WIRED4LIFE

My Journey to Becoming Wired

By: Dawn L. Huberty

DEDICATION

I dedicate this book to all wired people!

ACKNOWLEDGEMENTS

To God first; John 3:16.

My husband Jim Huberty and fur baby Max.

Ayenew, Woubeshet, Cardiologist at HCMC, Minneapolis
Jean C, Pacemaker Nurse at HCMC, Minneapolis

My parents for never giving up.

"For each new morning with its light,
For rest and shelter of the night,
For health and food, for love and friends,
For everything Thy goodness sends."
~Ralph Waldo Emerson

Contents

1. Introduction
2. Becoming Wired
3. Sharing Wired
4. The Evolution
5. Newsletter Archive
6. Sister Stories
   - A. Sandy
   - B. Amanda
   - C. Deb
   - D. Tay
   - E. Brenda
   - F. Diane
   - G. Fran
   - H. Nelly
   - I. Una
   - J. Mary Ellen
7. Wired Sister Visits
8. Facebook
9. Pets and Pacemakers
10. Warm Fuzzies
11. Wired Conferences
12. Mission Statement

13 Guest Contributors
14 Device Manufacturers
15 Encyclopedia
   A. What is a Pacemaker?
   B. What is an Implantable Cardioverter-Defibrillator?
   C. What is Heart Valve Disease?
   D. Common, everyday tests...
16 Laughter, the Best Medicine
17 Marian
18 WIRED4LIFE

INTRODUCTION

It appears from your tests that you have "third degree heart block with syncope." October 9, 1991. I heard these words for the first time. I finally had a diagnosis after 27 years. A pacemaker implant the next day and my wired journey began.

I cannot imagine for a moment what my life would look like without WIRED4LIFE being a large component. The women I've met, the experiences I've had, the knowledge I've gained, the overall feeling of wellness.

The idea for a WIRED4LIFE book was encouraged by many wired sisters and friends. I am starting with what I remember and what has been shared with me through the years. I pray you find your story here too.

BECOMING WIRED

My mother described the day of my baptism as one of fear and joy. Dad was driving the three of us to church for the first religious ritual of my young life. Mother, holding me, was sitting in the front seat of the car, next to dad. All of a sudden my head fell backwards and my body went limp. My mother yelled at dad to stop the car. As soon as this episode began, it ended. I was cooing and cuddling against my mother. I imagine their hearts then resumed a normal beat, as mine did. It was not the first and would not be the last time that I lost consciousness momentarily and immediately regained it. That day forward began 26 years of doctor appointments to try and determine why I had chronic fainting spells.

Among the many "conclusions" made by various doctors were that I would outgrow the fainting spells, that I was fainting 'for attention' or because I had bouts of constipation. All three were to prove incorrect.

Cod liver oil was prescribed, various vitamins and supplements, and specialists were called and seen, but a legitimate diagnosis was never made until the age of 27.

If you had looked through the window of my childhood, you would have seen many times when I was inactive, my nose buried in a book, the last to be picked for sports or neighborhood fun. It was primarily because I had no energy; the constant fainting spells were continuing to weaken my heart.

My mother died from breast cancer in 1978, it was a pivotal point in my young life and I always felt bad that she never knew that I did receive a proper diagnosis after battling much more than a "childhood ailment." My dad lived to see my first pacemaker implant; he died two years later.

From childhood into teenage years and then into my twenties, the fainting spells continued, but there was no reason why. It was my constant prayer that I would not be near people if I were to have a fainting spell because it was so embarrassing. I couldn't explain why it happened and it was easier to just wave it off, like it was no big thing.

The year I turned 26 I began fainting almost every day, and sometimes several times a day. I was having multiple tests, including scans of my brain; the most incomplete diagnosis at that time was that I was in the early stages of epilepsy, yet I had never had one symptom that was listed under the epilepsy umbrella.

I was given the option of further testing and/or medication. I chose neither and continued on with my life. I was learning to live with this disability. I had stopped driving, and even stopped taking the bus, because I knew when I would faint. I would occasionally have a five or ten second warning, and would see stars in the corner of my eyes, but all that would do was help prevent a terrible fall. Throughout the years of living with these fainting spells I had more than one black eye, or injury to my face, head or body.

In early October of 1991, after a year of continuous fainting spells with no diagnosis, I was spending the afternoon with my then mother-in-law and nephew. We were playing cards in the kitchen. I knew I had hit the floor, as I remember the fall, but for the first time ever, I was unable to speak. My nephew Billy hollered to his grandma that I had fallen and to please come into the kitchen. I was unresponsive and in order to expedite the process, my mother-in-law drove me to the hospital instead of calling for an ambulance. I regained consciousness by the time we arrived at Hennepin County Medical Center (HCMC) in Minneapolis, but felt exhausted. For the very first time in my entire life, I was hooked up to a heart monitor. An episode almost immediately was recorded on the device. A flurry of activity in the emergency room caused me to panic; I didn't realize it was me, at the center of the activity. But I was also extremely relieved that it was me; that at last, someone was taking me seriously, maybe someone was going to fix me.

Fix me, they did. After two days of rather intensive tests including 'tilt table', 'stress' and multiple blood work, it was determined that a lifetime of 'fainting spells' were now officially titled as 'third degree heart block (or complete heart block) with syncope' (fainting).

Basically, my heart was stopping each time I fainted. From that early episode at the age of a few months, until my 27th year of life, my heart had been stopping.

I was ecstatic at having a diagnosis, but petrified at the notion of having a pacemaker implanted inside my chest. It was a bittersweet day that I was told this would stop the fainting spells.

SHARING WIRED

In 2004 it was time to have a new pacemaker put in. Mine lasted 13 years, but as my cardiologist explained, pacemakers are like cars, do you want the newest model or an old beater? I decided the former was preferable! Who wants a beater pacemaker?

I was now 40 years old, I had moved past two decades with this device and along with a few gray hairs I also found myself in a state of anxiety. Worry had me thinking about the amount of time it would take to heal because I was older, what if this and that happened? I hopped on the internet and started obsessing about the "what-if's", unable to find help that didn't scare the pants off me.

I turned away from the internet and instead called my pacemaker nurse, Jean. I asked why there wasn't decent support (only fear induced postings), and she planted the seed in my head well before I ever had the surgery. "Why don't you start a group for women with pacemakers? You know a lot about your device, you are very educated as a patient and perhaps you will find someone like yourself." Say what??? Well I decided first things first, get the pacemaker put in and see how it all goes. Well, not that easy!

Prior to the pacemaker surgery I received a new diagnosis; a PFO (hole in my heart) was discovered from a TEE (transesophageal echocardiogram) test. I had experienced two different, and what I thought were unrelated events; two TIA's (mini strokes) in a period of four years. Each one left me unable to speak, move my body or communicate at all. Some testing was done, but determined nothing, so if "they" weren't worried, why should I be? I continued on.

It wasn't until my husband piped up during my pre-op appointment for the pacemaker, that I had in fact, had two these unusual events and how could I forget to tell them? Tests were done, and the decision was made to implant the pacemaker first, and a year later implant a septal occluder (patch) over both sides of the hole in my heart. Each surgery required the proper healing time.

If my anxiety levels were high before, now they were off the charts. I needed someone to talk to, I needed someone that was like me, a person without medical jargon to support and cheer me on. There was no one to be found. I could not find one person like me, not online, not through the many people I knew, and it left me feeling sad and empty. I couldn't be the only person out there who wished for a friend that could actually relate to some of the same heart issues.

WIRED4LIFE came from that need; a very personal need.

I started researching what was involved in starting a support group. I coined the phrase "WIRED4LIFE" after thinking purposely that the name needed to reflect the group as a whole. If you had a pacemaker, what was life like? What did it mean? Well, it most certainly meant you'd have it the remainder of your life. So you would be….wait for it…WIRED4LIFE. ☺ Since it was me that wanted to find a friend with similar heart conditions, I knew I had to start at the local level.

I posted ads in our newspaper, for a meeting every third Thursday. At the first meeting only two women showed up. One complained about the distance she had to travel and that she didn't think she needed support - while the other one (Marian) gushed that she was newly wired (a phrase I created with the name of the group) and was excited to see this group take off. At the second meeting, no one came; at the third meeting, Marian came back. At the 4th meeting when only Marian showed up again, we agreed to scrap the meetings and instead meet at Panera® around the corner for coffee & a visit. For 8 years Marian and I met for coffee and although she never understood how the internet worked, she gently prodded and pushed me to 'grow the group.' It was from this gentle prodding that I took the leap into the online world of support groups.

It started with a free Yahoo group, in which a few women took their own leap of faith into the group and continue, nine years later to be active & involved members.

These women joined in 2005 and are still actively involved!

Barbe'

Fran

Nelly

Janell

Jane

Janie

Sherry

Beckie

Nina

Two live in the United Kingdom, one, Canada, the rest are scattered throughout the U.S.

Initially we 'met' online each Saturday morning to chat. Oftentimes the subject went from our pacemakers to our grandchildren, but it was interesting getting to know each other. Unfortunately, there were a lot of burps with the Yahoo chat rooms back then, usually one or more of us would get kicked off, have to restart our computers and log back in. After a few years, the frustration level was so high; we only had one or two women in our weekly chat.

We tried another option, message boards instead of chat rooms, but it was still another place to have to log in. Most of our members were not internet or computer savvy, so the challenges continued.

We also had to deal with time zones. Our sisters on the east coast (1 hour later) or overseas (up to 6 hours later) were generally pretty open to meeting online at 8:30 a.m. CST, but our sisters to the west were not likely to join in at 6:30 or earlier on a Saturday morning. We made it work however, and into 2014, we still meet on the same day at the same time, except now we meet in a private Facebook group room!

In addition to a weekly chat, I began producing a semi-regular newsletter. At the time there were less than twenty sisters in the group, which was completely manageable for me. As we grew, the growing pains began. There were requests that we have midweek chats online, and if my work schedule allowed it, we would. I was still holding all the reigns of the group, so if I didn't set up the chat, no one was able to join in.

I relied heavily on a spreadsheet that helped me keep track of each member as they joined; it held their email address, implant date, name, contact info, joining date, birth date (oh yes, I had started recognizing birthdays in the newsletter and started sending an email-birthday card-as well), etc. This form of recording information served me well until a huge jump in membership.

We now had over 50 women who had found us from the various and many updates I made to our now 'free' website on Yahoo.

It was then I decided this little free group needed to become legitimate and official. I asked the women in the group if they would be willing to pay dues; $12 a year would help tremendously with the various bills that were accumulating and help toward implementing my idea for giving WIRED4LIFE proper status as an entity with the state of Minnesota. This way I could open a business checking account and use dues to pay expenses instead of it always coming out of my own pocket. This worked well for a number of years, WIRED4LIFE was able to support itself and I was learning all I could about creating and maintaining an online community.

In June 2006 I was approached by the magazine EP Lab Digest, "a product, news and clinical update for the electrophysiology professional." Mixed in with articles from St. Jude Medical and the American College of Cardiology Foundation was our first printed interview! "A Patient's Perspective: Living with a Pacemaker." I purposely discussed my own journey, which of course included the humble beginnings of WIRED4LIFE.

My introduction into printed media was what sprouted my love of writing and communication. I submitted snippets in the form of a monthly Q & A to Minnesota Women's Press, Minnesota Physician Publishing, Minnesota Health Care News, Minneapolis Star-Tribune and for my 'five minutes of national fame,' a letter to the editor of the now defunct BH&G Heart Healthy Living magazine, which did what I wanted it to do - brought new women into our group.

Wanting to reach a broader audience, I began writing regularly using the Yahoo 360 Blog program. I wrote about my own pacemaker journey, what being "wired" was like. In 2008 I began "Wired Words" with WordPress. I had written 260 posts with 153 recorded comments. For semi-regular blog posts, check out: https://wiredwords.wordpress.com

Marian and I were still meeting for coffee on a regular basis. She was notorious for not letting go of a certain subject. With each one, I tried to dismiss the subject by saying: "we simply do not have enough money." The first request from Marian was that we have our own pin. She would harp at me with the same conversation: "There is a Red Dress pin for women with heart disease; there are countless types of ribbons for various cancers or diseases. Why shouldn't we have our own pin?" Finally to quiet Marian, I did some research and found a company that would take our logo and create a pin. It was very expensive. I came to Marian with the quote and was sure that she would now, "let it go." Not only did she not 'let it go', she tried to convince me that it was the perfect timing to become nonprofit – and prodded me to fill out the paperwork and send in the fee-make it official.

If we were nonprofit we would have the money to not only to buy the pins (!!!), but also have conferences, bringing wired sisters together from across the globe to meet in person and learn more about their devices.

I researched; bought the dummy version of "How to Start a Non Profit." I read books, I talked to people who had traveled this path, and attended free workshops. From a distance it seemed doable. In a long phone call with Marian I told her I would attempt it, but made no promises. I didn't know if the sisters would step up to pay the $350 application fee and I didn't know if we would be approved. There was a lot more "not knowing" than knowing. What did I know about starting a nonprofit?

I initially knew nothing of starting an online support group either, but that worked out pretty good! There are no baby steps when you take a leap of faith such as this one. Each day I opened the mail to see checks from the wired sisters with encouraging notes cheering me on. First things first. I registered the name WIRED4LIFE with the state. I then assembled a group of people together to act as board members. And "act" wasn't too far from the truth. None of the assembled had any board experience, but alas, neither did I, so I figured we would wade the murky waters together.

With the 'sealed' documents in hand, I sent the application and check to the Internal Revenue Service. I said a quick prayer as I dropped it into the mail box; it was "Your will, not mine." This is how I live my life, so why should WIRED4LIFE be any different? WIRED4LIFE began as a need I had, but eventually blossomed into something much greater than my personal need. It became a community needed by many.

I was told the process could take 6-12 weeks. That is so darn vague. I waited and prayed. As I am known to do, I jumped the gun and scheduled our first board meeting. I figured "8 weeks out ought to be enough time." Miraculously, the official documentation arrived just DAYS before our first meeting. I breathed a great sigh of relief and sent out the congratulatory email to our wired sisters, sharing the good news. It was official; we were a 501(C)3 organization. I called Marian right away, she was ecstatic, always my cheerleader!

We had our first board meeting. As much delegating as I was able to do, the brunt of the work fell on me. I contacted the device manufacturers to submit grant applications and processed the endless paperwork and follow up that comes with being a nonprofit organization. We were now exactly that; an 'organization.'

What the money brought to our group was really quite wonderful. We ordered our own pins, we updated our outdated electronics (a new desktop computer with printer, updated software, even a smart phone). Business cards, magnets, and brochures were designed and ordered. We started planning our first WIRED4LIFE conference where 8 women took the opportunity to spend four days getting to know each other and learn about their devices.

We have since had four conferences and continue to have local get togethers and "lunch and learn" at both Medtronic and

Boston Scientific. We are planning a special conference in 2020, to celebrate the WIRED4LIFE 15th anniversary!

My own life was busy. I was working full-time, running a house filled with fur babies and a husband, dealing with the normal chores of life; laundry, cooking, cleaning.

From 2009-2012 I managed to handle everything myself without too much help from anyone else. As time went on, the parts that I loved about WIRED4LIFE were becoming smaller due to the constant 'book work'; the 'business' side had taken over and was starting to drain all of my good energy.

In 2012, I felt I had no other option than to give up our nonprofit status and become a 'not for profit' group. Most understood that I had gotten in deep, it was too much work for one person, and ultimately, they wanted me to be happy. I can report that now, I am!

All of this would have been different if I had brought on experienced board members in the beginning, hired an accountant and managed WIRED4LIFE as a nonprofit organization that was run like a business. But that was never my vision; the money was wonderful, greatly appreciated and we did good things with it, but in the end, I needed it to return to our roots.

I was planning our 3rd WIRED4LIFE conference, now named "gathering" for 18 women who were excited to learn about their devices and spend quality time with their sisters. We received our last grant request and the gathering came together nicely with help as always from the community of sisters.

Going forward I know there will be hiccups, but I am incredibly grateful that WIRED4LIFE has continued on from our humble beginnings in 2004, to hopefully many more years ahead.

On June 4, 2014 I received my third pacemaker implant. There were some issues, but I'm proud to say I'm the owner of a brand new shiny and much smaller Medtronic pacemaker!

THE EVOLUTION

What has continued to drive the need for WIRED4LIFE to grow and exist is the very basic need that all of us have; to be understood, heard and cared for. These are three incredible components to living life as a well-rounded human being.

WIRED4LIFE has evolved into a community, bigger than I could have ever imagined, but more importantly, a virtual coffee klatch where women get together with a cup of coffee and talk about life. We laugh, sometimes cry, and always support. We ask and answer questions. We cheer and hug. Not always virtually; how many women from across the globe have met in person, from the root of WIRED4LIFE?

There are offshoots all over Facebook; groups started by women who originally came from WIRED4LIFE. I feel like a proud grandmother, but am always a sister. A wired sister.

NEWSLETTER ARCHIVE

Here, a few snippets of past newsletters:

September 2004: "The FDA is trying to find ways to make MRI's safe for people with certain implants." (The reality is now that MRI compatible devices have been created and have been successfully implanted). Including MRI safe leads (wires). The unfortunate fact is that those of us with deeply embedded old leads (20 years or more) are ineligible for these type of devices. Lead extraction is more common, but is difficult and by some considered too risky. On a medical note, the PET (positron emission tomography) scan can be used safely with implanted devices.

May 2005: Regarding the 'thorn in my side' microwave question: Modern pacemakers are shielded from EMI (electromagnetic interference) by a backup mode that takes over if a really strong EMI disrupts the main circuits programming.

July 2005: Our membership base was at 21 and I was ecstatic! We had three wired sisters in Canada, 'a handful' from the west coast, the majority on the east coast and three in Minnesota!

Skipping ahead to March 2006: A common thread was coming together as I began to receive email and letters in the mail from new members. 1) Many of us had spent a big chunk of our life ill, undiagnosed, misdiagnosed and uncertain what exactly was wrong with us. And 2) the medical profession did not take our worries or concerns seriously. This created a flurry of activity in our chat room each week, what could "WE" do to better educate the doctors. I believed then, as I do now, it needs to start with the folks in ER or Urgent Care. It was a podiatrist doing his residency in Emergency who hooked me up to a heart monitor and right away the machine was beeping! That is always my personal joke: "a foot doctor found my heart disease."

WIRED4LIFE had been (and still is) a strong supporter of the **Go Red for Women** movement. They have been instrumental in educating all people; from nurses and doctors to the women themselves, that heart disease is not just a man's problem and that our symptoms are much different than men experience.

Part of what I hoped to accomplish with WIRED4LIFE was empowering the women in our group to share their stories with others, particularly their own family, as heart disease is often hereditary. The more you know, the better qualified you are to care for your own physical health.

As women are generally the center of their home and family, they are also often the last to be cared for. With WIRED4LIFE I wanted a very strong component of our community to be offering emotional support and friendship; a safety net, a place where women could gather together on the computer, on a phone call and in person. A conversation to have that made it clear: "you are not alone and there is someone like you in this group. We've been where you are and we are here to support."

Every few months I changed the format and design of the newsletter and received quite a few compliments! Some were noting the brightness and colors, an easier to read font, but always the content. The members were learning about their devices, and were now starting to ask questions.

For quite some time I shared 'healthy recipes' or tips. The January 2007 issue shows a yummy recipe for BBQ chicken salad, the next month, one for a bran-muffin breakfast trifle! We had our own website finally, www.wired4life.net, which is still in use today.

Education was particularly of interest to our members, and for me it was a chance to do research. With complete internet access it was more of a task to weed out incorrect information and make certain that what I was presenting was fact.

The three main device manufacturers; Medtronic, Boston Scientific and St. Jude Medical were more than willing to provide documentation through their own websites and answer occasional questions via email or the phone.

Learning about our devices and how they 'ticked' was probably the most often asked question. From there, the questions ran the gamut from battery life to what does the computer chip do? Why are magnets bad, what is EMI, etc.

We also have been incredibly blessed through the years to have members who were also cardiac nurses. One such sister, Jill Flatt, wrote her own column titled "Ask-A-Nurse." Questions were asked and she answered in a way that we could understand (non-medical terminology) and also educated us on the various procedures or specifications that we wanted to learn.

For many years we were a group devoted to providing support for sisters with cardiac pacemakers only.

A member with a pacemaker ended up with an upgrade to a defibrillator. This was unchartered territory, I didn't really understand what a defibrillator did in comparison to a pacemaker. It was another learning curve, but one I felt was important that we consider supporting; both educationally and emotionally. One of the biggest differences is that a defibrillator 'shocks' or 'delivers therapy,' unlike a pacemaker which most of the time we are not aware is even working.

One more addition came in 2009, when we opened the door to women with replacement heart valves. These were now the three primary implanted cardiac devices that we would continue to provide education and support for.

It was at this point that we could no longer consider ourselves a small coffee klatch, we were now reaching across the globe with outstretched wired arms.

When the idea for this book came to light, many of the women were not only anxious to share their story, but many wanted to add an updated version.

As I believe that WIRED4LIFE is a community of women, this book would not make any sense if it didn't include the path taken by our sisters; to becoming wired.   I am greatly appreciative for all who have shared their journey with us.

SISTER STORIES

When I began the newsletter in 2005 I regularly interviewed members to share their story. The newsletters themselves were a wonderful tool for communication. I researched and shared pertinent information regarding our implanted devices, do's and don'ts, how to best care for yourself when you are the primary caregiver, etc. And, of course that topic that comes up time and time again, is a microwave unsafe for our devices? This is one question that always gives me fits!

There are many excerpts from past newsletters that are still valuable and need to be shared, rather than locked up on a flash drive. The beautiful thing about writing a book is that it will stand the test of time. It can be a tool for generations to come.

The very first woman to share her story was **Rose**, who lived in a small farming community in North Central Illinois. We have since been in touch, and her most recent update is:

"You are writing a book!? Awesome! Update on me? Nothing much has changed, pacemaker wise. I'm on my 2nd pacer and have 3 years left on its life now. I just continue to be thankful there is such a thing as pacemakers as I know I would have croaked long before now, without it.

For many years I did the phone check of the pacer. That was very irritating. I should say the people that did the phone checks were very irritating. They treated me like I must be 95 years old and no brain in my head. And I usually got a rep that didn't speak English and then acted like there was something wrong with me because I couldn't understand them. I vented at one of my in office pm checks and was told I could just do it in their office every 3 months. Much better! At last check the Medtronic rep said my own heartbeat is 30 bpm…enough to keep me alive but I wouldn't feel well."

Individual wired sister stories have not been edited.

Sandy

Hello Wired Sisters! My name is Sandy Overeem and I will be married to my wonderful husband Robert for 25 years this coming summer!

I have 1 daughter – Elizabeth who just turned 30! She is married to a great man and they have 1 child – Mikey. Mikey just turned 1 in February and we just LOVE being grandparents! My husband and I live in Lake Hopatcong, NJ with 6 crazy cats. I have had "Darla" my St. Jude Medical Vic-tory 5816 pacemaker since December 2008. It was an adjustment but I am truly thankful for 'Darla' my trusted pacemaker. My quality of life has certainly improved and I wear her as a badge of honor.

I grew up in Brooklyn, NY and I was not a particularly active kid; never had any stamina for running or things like that and I really didn't give it much thought. I could do normal stuff and walked a lot but would get a bit breathy on hills or if I ran. In hind-sight I wonder if these were just symptoms that were never detected.

I had my daughter at a fairly young age (I was just under 21). I was engaged to her biological father but kept stalling on marriage. Smart move on my part and before she was two I finally wised up and cut him from our lives. Let's just say it was not a healthy relationship for me and certainly not for my daughter. Fortunately a couple of years later I met a wonderful man. We had actually gone to junior high school together and had some mutual friends – but we don't remember each other. It was a whirlwind romance. We met (again) in the summer of 1986 and were married in Holland the following sum-mer. During most of that time we lived in 2 different countries.

I worked for a printer for 10 years. I left there after tragedy truck my family. My sister's middle son was killed – by a friend. It was a horrible time for our family and in many ways my sister has still not recovered. I left work to be able to be there through the trial. It is a long story and still baffles me today…..it comes down to two lives lost. My sister will never get her son back and the other boy is still in jail. His life ended that day too.

After all that I did not want to have a high pressure job. So I decided to be a temp. That didn't last long as one company was looking to hire me; a small furniture importer and I ended up working there for over ten years. When the owner retired at the end of 2008, a few employees; including myself, decided to buy him out and now we have our own company!

Ironically it was at the end of 2008 that my health turned for the worse. My commute from New Jersey to NYC involved a lot of walking to and from trains and up and down subway stairs.

I had been noticing that sometimes when I got to the stop of the stairs – which I had been doing for years – I couldn't breathe. I kept assuming it was because of my weight but I would lose a couple of pounds and it would be a bit better, but some days it would be there and I would have to stop and catch my breath, as time went on, I just ignored it.

Finally one day in November 2008 I went up the stairs in my house to get ready for bed. I walked fast but was not running and when I got the top, I almost collapsed. My husband kept saying are you ok? I couldn't talk but nodded my head for yes (stubborn me...) Do we need to go to the emergency room? Shake head no! Maneuver myself to the bed and sit. Catch breath - husband still worried. I say – that was weird, I have never had that happen before. Husband – let's go to the emergency room. Me: NO I'll call doctor in morning. Must be allergies or maybe I am getting asthma or something.

Well it did scare me and I did go to my primary the next day. I was pushing the exercise/asthma theory but my doctor is very good and said – cardiologist first then we will look at other theories. So off I go to make an appointment with the cardiologist – Dr. Z. He listened to everything I had to say, did an EKG and an echo, didn't see much but based on what I said happened, ordered a Holter monitor.

Now he did mention the possibility of needing a pacemaker and explained the whole 'electrical short' as being like a lamp with a loose wire. Sometimes it lights, sometimes it doesn't. I did a lot of nodding as I was now suffering from 'Deer in the Headlight Syndrome!" I was hooked up to the monitor (I don't even remember how long I had to wear it) and left with an appointment for the day after Thanksgiving for a stress test. I got to my car and it all sank in. I dialed my husband at work and then the tears started and I don't even think he could understand a word I said, but fortunately he has a lot of patience and was able wait until I cried

It was only about a week later, the day of the stress test finally arrived. They hooked me up and started the treadmill and as Dr. Z. looked at the screen and watched the beats; beat to skip, 1 skip, 2 skip, 3 skip, 4. I have never seen anyone stop a treadmill so fast. He turned to me and said "You've never passed out???" No I hadn't.

Back in the exam room we reviewed everything again and he explained more about the pacemaker. He said we don't want to skip the forest for the trees. Even though my blood pressure and cholesterol were all good he wanted to schedule a heart catherization. We were able to schedule it for before Christmas – I wanted it over with. He did tell me that if it was all clear I would need to meet the EP (Dr. C.) and discuss the pacemaker further. Dr. Z did go into detail about how it worked and what it would be like.

The cath was scheduled for December 17th and all was clear. (The worst thing for me, was having to lie down for all of those hours after). I was still lying down in the hospital when Dr. C the EP came over to see me. He was great, he sat and talked with me and my husband and explained it all. Then he said it was up to me but since I was there he could do it the next day or I could schedule it for after the holidays. I really didn't want to have this hanging over my head for that long and I was scared so I said let's do it tomorrow. After a cardiac MRI to rule out anything else we did.

That would have been fine except when I came out of the pacemaker surgery and was put in my room I freaked out. I think it all finally sank in. I was also feeling a 'thumping 'in my chest, a bit painful but more annoying. I asked why I had chest pain (not incision pain) when I never had it before. My husband turned white – I think this was harder on him than on me in some ways. Chest x-ray time (I had lots of those). They thought it was just hitting my diaphragm and told me to wait till morning (surgery was at around 5 pm) so it wasn't such a long time to wait.

The next morning they came in and explained that they wanted to test me for Brugada Syndrome as they saw some-thing to indicate that I might have to trade my pacemaker for a DEFIBRILLATOR. I had to go back for a special EKG with a dye. The good news was that they are 99% sure that I don't have it.
(Doctors will never say 100! Lol) But they did say that a lead shifted and I might have to have it redone – they were trying for later that day but I had already eaten breakfast and lunch. It was snowing heavily that day and I had sent my husband home. The 30 minute drive home from the hospital took my husband over 2 hours. They decided to do the surgery in the late afternoon. My husband wanted to come back to the hospital but I didn't want to

worry about him on the roads. The doctor promised to call him as soon as I was done. This time everything worked out well.

I was finally able to go home the next day. I was very nervous about using my left arm. I am left-handed and so it is an instinct to use that arm. Although they didn't tell me to, I had read online that many people slept in a sling. I opted to do that the first few days as many times I would shoo a cat away with that arm. When I went back the following week they told me not to worry about it. I did what they said but I was still nervous! My family was worse than I was; it was sit down, don't do that, I'll get that. Now I knew what I couldn't do, but I was still able to do certain things.

In the middle of this we were closing the office in NY and moving computers to our homes and setting up a new company, plus there was Christmas shopping to be done and I couldn't drive for a while but I managed to get most of it done.

It took me awhile to get moving only because in the middle of all this I had torn my Achilles tendon and had to wear this boot-thing for 3 months. It was difficult to get around and so I kept my factory settings for a while. It wasn't till almost a year later when I was working on losing weight, doing a lot of walking that I noticed that I was still out of breath on hills. It certainly wasn't as bad as before the pacemaker but my heart rate still didn't go up. I was diagnosed with 2nd Degree Heart Block Mobitz. I was told that my heart rate during normal standing/sitting/ sleeping and mild movement was ok, but when I exercised it would drop. Since heart rate monitors don't usually work with a pacemaker I ordered a pulse oximeter. This allowed me to carry it when I was walking and get a reading on my heart rate. It would only go up from 60 to around 100 or 105. (They like to save battery life!).

I did a lot of research online about settings and brought my findings along with my cur-rent settings to my doctor. He understood what I was saying but ordered a stress test to make sure nothing else was going on. He called my EP and advised him of the findings. The EP agreed with my research and advised we could skip the stress test and just reprogram. I spent a long time with the technician changing settings and having me run around the hospital up and down stairs and then again and again until we got it right. I now can pace to 150 and it will track my heart rate to 160. I can finally exercise – oh those hills sometimes get to me but now I see improvement when I am outside hiking on a regular basis. Now I am at the point that my breathlessness is truly from a need to be in better shape.

It was during my research on pacemakers and settings that I found WIRED4LIFE. I will honestly say that initially I didn't join as it was a 'pay' group. I had been visiting another group that is free but there was a lot of politics and while researching the posts could be helpful, the site seemed to have an almost high school environment – there was definitely an 'in crowd'. I never felt like I belonged. There was a lot of technical information which for me, in the beginning, was needed. I like to know how things work and it allowed me to find a list of questions to bring to my doctor with questions, but I grew out of that fast.

Then I decided that I liked the idea of a group of women supporting each other. WIRED4LIFE has a much different feel. I'm still quiet most of the time, but I don't feel like there is an 'in crowd'. Everyone is 'IN'. Everyone is equal and welcome.

This group isn't something you 'grow out of' it is a community of women that is evolving and growing and is there for each other no matter what. It is truly special and that is because Dawn is special and each of you are as well.

We are fortunate to live at a time where first of all we have these crazy contraptions that can save our lives and in many cases improve them and that we live in this digital world where we can connect with people from all over and support each other.

Amanda

I am a small town girl, born and raised in a town of less than 2500 people and 30 miles away from the nearest Wal-Mart or decent grocery store. It is there that I met my husband Barkley. We were high school sweethearts and married 6 months after I graduated high school. We have a Boxer we call 'H' and 2 cats. One is a rescue kitty, her name is Libby and the other is Mowgli, a Bengal.

Our marriage started out a bit bumpy when 10 days before our wedding, Barkley had a motorcycle accident. He was released from the hospital on the day of our wedding, and despite the fact that he was in a hospital bed and heavily medicated, we got married…in my in-law's living room. It wasn't the dream wedding I had planned, but it was quite the celebration.

Since that time, we have put our vows of "in sickness and in health" to the test. The true trial began when at the age of 23; I was diagnosed with heart disease. As a young woman, I had my fair share of headaches, but I noticed during that summer that my headaches were becoming much more frequent and bothersome. Over-the-counter medications proved useless so I sought help from my family physician. He prescribed everything from migraine medications to prescription strength pain killers, assuming it was just a headache. Nothing eased the pain and within a few weeks of the onset of my headaches, I experienced my first fainting episode.

I remember waking up dazed and confused, on the floor of our entry way, with my husband standing over me. While getting ready for work that morning, I had lost consciousness. We called the doctor, who saw me immediately; then the testing began. I was checked for brain tumors, diabetes, and a slew of other medical conditions, with my heart being last on the list. After all other testing had been exhausted my doctor referred me to a cardiologist on the slim chance that my heart was the culprit.

My first cardiologist was an older, distinguished looking gentleman, who assured me that we would get to the bottom of all this. He immediately ordered an EKG, an echocardiogram, and a carotid artery scan. The echo did reveal some slight abnormalities, but still nothing that would explain my fainting episodes. I left his office with a 48 hour Holter monitor, in hopes of finding out what was going on.

In usual fashion, while wearing the monitor I had only very minor symptoms and no fainting episodes. This prompted my cardiologist to do a tilt table test. I was sent to the hospital for this test, where all sorts of monitors were put on me and an IV was placed in my arm. I was strapped to a table lying down and was then gradually tilted up to a standing position. I was given drugs to challenge my system, but the doctor was unable to provoke an episode. Even though I did not faint, my heart rate and blood pressure did not respond appropriately. My cardiologist knew we were on the right track and referred me to one of his colleagues, an Electrophysiologist.

I met with this new specialist and was immediately comforted by her warm disposition and willingness to listen. She did a second tilt table test and scheduled an EP study for the following week. This was the first time that I had ever been admitted to the hospital and I was frightened. I remember bits and pieces of the procedure, as I was only slightly sedated and still somewhat conscious. Again, this test did not reveal the cut and dry answers that we were looking for, so an implantable loop recorder was placed in my chest. It is a small device implanted in the chest that continuously records heart activity for up to two years. Being the over-achiever that I am, I fainted within the first 10 days of receiving the device. I don't think I had ever been so happy to fall flat on my face, at least now they would have the evidence on the monitor and everyone would know that I wasn't crazy!

During my post-op follow up appointment my loop recorder was interrogated for the first and only time. A representative Medtronic hooked me up to her computer and asked questions pertaining to my episodes. I was surprised to find out that the recorder picked up not only the episode that I recorded when I fainted, but it had also recorded several episodes that I was completely unaware of. She printed out several pages of information and told me she would discuss the findings with my doctor and they would be back shortly to talk to me.

After what felt like an eternity of waiting, I excused myself to the bathroom. Of course, when I got back to the exam room my doctor, nurse, and the device rep were all waiting for me.

The somber look on each of their faces said it all. My doctor proceeded to tell me that the findings had revealed my heart rate had gotten dangerously slow numerous times and had even stopped at one point. She gently informed me that I needed a pacemaker and I needed it soon. She gave me an option, but said it had to be done by the end of the week.

I took the news well and held my composure until my husband and I left her office. As soon as we walked out of the door though, I cried my eyes out. I'm still not sure if it was because I was terrified to have surgery or relieved to finally have an answer.

On November 23, 2007, the day after Thanksgiving, I received my first pacemaker. The surgery went perfectly and I was discharged the following day. My arm was in a sling to remind me not to lift my arm above shoulder level, but I was so sore that I didn't need much help remembering. I took it easy for the first two weeks and by the New Year I was feeling pretty good; the fainting had stopped and I tried to get back to life as usual. Physically I was fine, but I was having a hard time wrapping my head around the fact that I had a pacemaker in my early 20's.

Every twinge and funny feeling in my chest had me panicking; I thought that life would never be the same.

In an effort to reassure myself that this was all normal, I turned to the internet and stumbled upon WIRED4LIFE. I was overjoyed; an on-line support group for women with pacemakers! Without hesitation I joined the group and was embraced by a sister-hood of women who had all been where I was. There is never a question too silly or request too insignificant. We reach out to each other in times of joy and happiness or in times of fear and insecurity. We all share one common bond that makes us sisters for life…our wired hearts.

No matter what, my wired sisters have been there for me every step of the way. For me, getting a device was just the beginning of my journey. It turns out that a slow heart rate wasn't the only problem with my heart. I was plagued with other arrhythmias and host of complications not related to my device that have necessitated intervention. I have required several ablations, two open heart surgeries, numerous pacemaker surgeries and have battled two life threatening infections. In total I have endured over 25 heart-related surgeries and procedures and my doctors are certain that at some point I will require another open-heart surgery in addition to the surgeries required to keep up with my pacemaker.

By no means is my journey complete; I am still traveling this road we call heart disease. I am only alive today thanks to an incredible God and amazing advancements in technology. A small recording device helped diagnose me and my heart beats today thanks to an intricate piece of technology called a pacemaker.

One thing is for sure though; I am both a medical mystery and a medical miracle. My greatest lesson has been to ALWAYS listen to your body and NEVER lose hope. Through it all my faith in God has seen me through and I know without a doubt that God must have a pretty special plan for my life, because He's been working overtime to keep me here.

Deb

My story starts in 1955 when I was born with a ventricular septal defect (a hole in my heart). We lived in Toronto at the time and my parents were told that Sick Kids wasn't having the success that they were in the states so we headed down to the Mayo Clinic in Rochester, MN in 1957. Their success rate was 50/50. I was one of the lucky ones, but went into heart block shortly afterwards.....finally going home 3 months after surgery with a heartbeat of 44 beats per minute. I was 2 years old.

From the age of 2-9 I had several heart spells when my heart would slow to 17 b/m or actually stop – lucky for me my dad was there that time, to get me beating again whilst waiting for the ambulance. Stressful time for them for sure!

In 1964 Dr. William Mustard, at Sick Kids, told my folks that they had this fairly new "implantable" pacemaker that they were having some success with, in kids like me with heart block. So, at the age of 9, I had my first pacemaker implanted in my abdomen. It was a success and two weeks later I went home (two WEEKS!!! Compare that to the overnight stay that I now have for any new ones!).

In three years, I'd outgrown my leads (that were actually stitched onto the heart) and they broke…so rather than stitch more on, they swung the pacemaker up under my left arm which is where it was for the next 3 years (not the most comfortable location!).

After that, it was then situated on my left chest, but it slid down into my left breast where the next several pacemakers resided. Personally, I liked it there! I could wear a bikini and it was hidden...my original open heart surgery scar was horizontal, not vertical as they are today so you couldn't see it. The only scar that showed was the one in my abdomen – and for a teen THAT was GREAT!

The down side to those old pacemakers was the fact that they didn't change rate. Once it was set at 72 beats a minute it was ALWAYS 72 beats a minute. This could be the reason for me developing heart failure later in life – about 13 years ago. But once again technology stepped in and 7 years ago I had my first bi-ventricular pacemaker/defibrillator implanted on the right side, after they lasered out several of my old leads. Since then my heart failure has improved a whole "class"...I feel better...have more energy and my EF that was less than 20 is now 32! I am on my second bi-ventricular unit and going strong! I have 2 children and 5 grandchildren and a golden retriever. I also have two younger sisters that have NO heart problems. My husband and I winter in Florida (I like to say that's one of the perks of heart failure – getting out of our Ontario winters!!!)...we now live at our cottage by Lake Huron. Life is GOOD!

What I'd like to finish off with here girls is this...your attitude is your biggest asset (or liability of course)...be happy, enjoy your family and your friends. Take comfort in knowing that you're not alone – my goodness what DID we do before Facebook?

That has been a huge plus in my life. I've met two others who have had pacemakers almost as long as I have – they both got theirs in 1967, three years after I did. It's been great comparing stories! And then joining Wired4Life and now planning on meeting you all at a future conference is the icing on the cake!

So for those of you that are just starting out on this journey, take heart! With technology and meds today we can live a happy life…maybe a bit more sedate than most, but you know…it sure beats the alternative!

Tay

Hello, my name is Tay; I live in Kuwait and have been an active member of WIRED4LIFE since 2006. The time had finally come, it was October 1979, I was 23 years old and about to undergo open heart surgery to correct the anomalous drainage of two superior pulmonary veins and the atrial septal defect (ASD) I had been dealing with since birth. Being born with ASD, I suffered through many seizures and fainting spells during my childhood.

I was promised that with the successful completion of this surgery, I would have a new life to look forward to, one in which I would no longer suffer minute to minute from shortness of breath, or unannounced black outs. I was anxious, but eager to see the outcome. Thankfully, the cardiologists proved to be correct as after the surgery I felt a vast improvement in my ability to breath and finally began living my life like any other individual in my peer group would.

I got married, had three wonderful children, and worked on building a home.

Nearly ten years later in 1989, as my husband and I had begun settling in Kuwait, I started noticing that my pulse rate would drop and I began fainting quite frequently again.

When I consulted my cardiologist he informed me that I would need a pacemaker. Unfortunately Kuwait at that time was not equipped with pacemakers or the appropriate professionals to perform the procedure. Because of this on July 17th, 1990 I was sent to Memphis, TN to have a double chamber pacemaker installed.

The surgery was a success and I returned to Kuwait on July 30th only to be victim to an invasion by the Iraqis two days later. Thankfully, I had completed the surgery before the war, and had returned in time to be with my family and flee from the dangers of war back to Tennessee where I continued to receive treatment.

After the war was over we moved back and resettled in Kuwait. Eight years had passed at this point and I was beginning to feel faint. I woke up one morning in a deep sweat and felt a severe pain in my chest. I was dizzy and knew something wasn't right, so I drove myself to the hospital, which in retrospect was very, very dumb.

I was immediately admitted and told that just after 8 years my battery had worn out and I was in need for a replacement pacemaker. Since my health care providers could not find a double chamber device, they instead decided to use a used single chamber pacemaker that was available.

The cardiologist attempted to attach the new pacemaker to the old leads that were already present in my chest from the first surgery. Unfortunately he was unable to do this and instead opted to create a new incision on the other side of my chest and put the new leads in on that side. Thankfully I survived the surgery, but did not feel right; I was still having palpitation problems. When I discussed this with my cardiologist he assured me that this was a normal side effect and offered me medication to treat it.

Finally by 2004 Kuwait had a full-fledged pacemaker specialist working in the country and I approached her complaining of the palpitation, shortness of breath I had been experiencing. She suggested that I undergo yet another procedure where she would replace my single chamber pacer with that of a double. I agreed and had the procedure done.

After this, my fourth surgery, I was still feeling as if something had not been done correctly. I still was feeling miserable and couldn't understand why I was not feeling significantly better after surgery. Deciding to do my own research I went on the net and started posting my concerns on various pacemaker support sites. It was then that I discovered Dawn and WIRED4LIFE. As soon as I posted my question Dawn immediately responded, offering answers, help, and mere acknowledgment that issues such as mine were being shared by many more than I knew.

With the full support of my WIRED4LIFE sisters in 2006 I went for my fifth pacemaker change in which the cardiologist attempted to insert another lead for me to have a double chamber pacemaker. Unfortunately this cardiologist's attempts were unsuccessful and she informed me that I would need to have some of the leads removed by laser so that there could be enough space for her to add a new lead for the replacement device. Since the operation was very risky (I was informed in my case that there was a less than 10% survival rate) and the technology was not readily available in Kuwait my case got forwarded to the Cleveland Clinic.

Upon my arrival at the clinic, the pacemaker technician who looked at my reports looked dumbfounded. He said; 'it's no wonder you've been suffering with palpitations, extreme exhaustion and a whole slew of complications, you have been wired incorrectly!'

I came to find out that instead of having my upper ventricle pacing they had me pacing in the lower ventricle. Apparently during all these years from 1998 until 2006 each of the many pacemaker procedures that had been done, were repeating this same mistake which was causing my heart to enlarge along with numerous other complications. I now felt somewhat relieved that my concerns were validated, but anxious at the course of action necessary to correct it.

On September 6th, 2006 as I was being wheeled into surgery I said my final goodbyes to my husband and children. Knowing the risks involved with laser surgery, I was nervous, but calmed down significantly when I reminisced on all the wonderful things that I had seen and people I had met. Knowing that I was in a circle of prayers from Dawn and all my wired sisters eased my worries and before I knew it I was out, resting, at peace. Suddenly, as if I was snapped up by the neck I was pulled back and opened my eyes to see my doctor telling me everything was over, he said he managed to insert another lead in the artery and avoided the laser procedure entirely and I now had a fully functioning double chamber Medtronic pacemaker.

I was thrilled and after seeing my family's faces again I immediately wanted to get word out to Dawn and all my wired sisters that I was ok and that I could feel their prayers during surgery. Had it not been for the hope and love shown to me by all you wonderful women, I would have never entered surgery with such poise and calm.

The countless support you lovely ladies at WIRED have offered is immeasurable. I am thrilled that such a wonderful group exists and am even more excited and proud to call myself a member. God Bless you all!!!

Brenda

My grandparents were very healthy and lived a long life. My maternal grandfather reminded me of Jack Lalanne. He exercised every morning and took long walks in the neighborhood and on the beach in Florida where he and my grandmother lived. Conversely, I never knew my paternal grandfather because he died of a heart attack when my dad was a teenager. My paternal grandmother died of a stroke when she was 76 and I was eleven years old.

In keeping with the family history, my father had his first heart attack when he was 51 but it was mild and he had little damage. After his second, more serious heart attack, I rushed back from Germany where my family was living at the time to be by his side when he underwent quadruple bypass surgery. In the ten years following, he had two more heart attacks, one more bypass surgery and a diagnosis of congestive heart failure for which he needed a pacemaker to prolong his life. I always hoped I would take after my mother's side but feared I would end up with heart disease in middle age. My fears came true, but from the most unlikely source.

In 1985 while living in Germany with my husband and young daughter I suddenly started having severe heart palpitations.

I went to see a doctor who said he couldn't detect anything and it would probably pass. But it didn't pass. The symptoms appeared periodically and continued for years with no diagnosis. With no evidence of disease and one doctor after another telling me I was fine, I began to think I was losing my mind.

My symptoms grew more severe in the early 2000's so I started the hunt again for a doctor who would listen and help me figure out what was wrong. After a stress test showed nothing, one cardiologist actually told me that if I just stopped thinking about it the symptoms would go away. I went to my car and cried for a half hour, convinced that I would never know what was wrong with me. In the mid-2000's, I was lucky enough to find a new, wonderful and caring, primary care physician. When I told her that I had been dealing with these troublesome heart rhythm symptoms for so many years and I desperately wanted to find a cardiologist who could help, she recommended I find an electrophysiologist. I had never even heard of this type of doctor before. She said that an electrophysiologist is a specialist for heart rhythm issues (electrical vs plumbing). I was hopeful that I would find some answers.

By the time I found an electrophysiologist and got an appointment, I was so fatigued that I had trouble going to work each day. He was very understanding, took his time asking me about my symptoms and explained his thoughts about the possible issues I was dealing with.
He arranged for me to have a 24-hour halter monitor, but as luck would have it I didn't have any heart palpitations during that time. I thought he'd give up on me at that point, but he said he wanted to do a 7-day halter monitor that was designed to allow

me to record only when there was an episode. During that week, I had several episodes. When I had my follow-up with him he said, "I have some answers." I was so relieved. He explained that every single time I recorded an episode (60+ times) the monitor picked up moderate to severe Premature Ventricular Contractions (PVC's). Finally!!

He recommended daily high doses of Magnesium Malate (and some other supplements – no drugs) to manage the symptoms. He was right. I took the supplements he recommended and was soon relieved of almost all of the PVC's that had plagued me for so many years. In the back of my mind, however, I couldn't shake the feeling that there was something else going on.

In the spring of 2009, I became very ill with flu symptoms, dizziness, severe fatigue and fainting spells. I was hospitalized overnight for observation and sent home the next day. The dizziness and fatigue continued, but the fainting subsided for two years. Then in 2011, the fainting returned. My husband took me to the ER where the ER doc witnessed and was able to monitor my heart rate during repeated fainting spells.

The diagnosis was Sick Sinus Syndrome and the remedy was a pacemaker. I was shocked and confused and wanted nothing to do with a pacemaker. The docs told me that if I didn't agree to a pacemaker I would lose my driving privileges. My very patient husband finally convinced me to get the pacemaker by pointing out that I could faint while carrying a grandbaby or driving a car with them in it and harm them (or myself or others on the road).

My pacemaker surgery was on a very memorable day - Cinco de Mayo (May 5) 2011. I would have much preferred to be at a party eating chips and guacamole. Instead, I was in the hospital having leads inserted into my heart and a pacemaker into my chest. I was convinced this was the beginning of the end for me and I'd soon have heart attacks and bypass surgery just like my dad. After a while I realized that things could have been much worse. The pacemaker saved my life. I went from resenting it to appreciating it and being very thankful for such amazing technology.

At my 3-month follow-up, I asked my electrophysiologist if he knew why this had happened to me. What caused Sick Sinus Syndrome? He asked me a strange question – he said, "have you ever been bitten by a tick." I told him I had – my friends and family used to go camping when I was a teenager and I liked to hike, had dogs, etc. I had suspected Lyme disease years earlier but was told by my previous primary doctor that there was no way I had Lyme because I didn't have joint pain. I couldn't believe my ears. I had no idea that Lyme disease could damage your heart.

He suggested I learn more about Lyme disease and find a Lyme Literate Doctor (LLMD) to explore the possibility that I might have been infected with Lyme disease and/or other co-infections for years. In my quest for information about Lyme, I learned that current testing is very unreliable and often has false negative results. The tests do not detect Lyme disease in your blood. They look for antibodies that your body produces when it is infected with Lyme disease. But Lyme is a tricky disease and cleverly hides in something called biofilm to avoid being killed off, so the antibodies may not even be active at the time of the test even if you are infected with the disease. Patients have much better outcomes when they are diagnosed and treated early (within three months) before it is considered chronic. My LLMD diagnosed me by using a combination of blood test results and symptom assessment, the same way you would a number of other diseases that have no reliable blood test.

If you think you or a loved one may have been infected with Lyme, don't wait. Find a Lyme Literate MD as soon as possible. If you found the tick that bit you, DO NOT DESTROY IT! Carefully remove it (do not use nail polish, just pull it straight up and out with a tweezer – slowly and carefully) and place it in a plastic zipper sandwich bag and seal it, then place it inside another and seal it. Contact your local health department to see if they offer free testing to see if the tick is carrying Lyme disease.

There are countless online resources about Lyme disease, but be careful. There are always those who would take advantage of someone who is desperate for help. A couple of resources I've found that are especially helpful:

www.lymedisease.org - has a plethora of research articles and publishes an electronic magazine called, "Lyme Times," with helpful articles and information on everything from how to remove a tick to the details about Lyme disease and co-infections. They also solicit information from patients and providers to gather data about the real effects of Lyme disease – look for MyLymeData on their webpage.

www.natcaplyme.org – the National Capital Lyme Disease Association is based in the Washington D.C. Metropolitan area. They provide information on public policy and behind the scenes issues affecting your access to care and treatment. They also have regional support groups and information about how to find care and support across the country.

I have tried to look for the good that came from this experience. For me, it has demonstrated the need to always be true to yourself and your instincts. Don't ever let anyone in the medical community dismiss your concerns. If you feel that you haven't been heard, find another practitioner and insist on receiving the care you deserve. Keep looking until you find the right fit so that you can remain as healthy as possible throughout your life.

I continue to thrive despite my chronic Lyme disease and at least two co-infections. I count my blessings every day and among them my three grandchildren who will probably never know how much they mean to me. I remind them with hugs and love every time I see them. There are three main components in my life that help me stay healthy. First, the unfailing support of my wonderful, kind, patient and understanding husband who has been by my side and has been my rock through every bit of this crazy ride. I also have an amazing LLMD who is always open to hearing my concerns and willing to work with me to tailor my care around my needs. And finally, I continue to work full time and am grateful every day that I have health insurance to cover most of my medical expenses. Medical care should not be a privilege reserved only for those who are healthy enough to work or wealthy enough to pay.

My hope is that researchers will develop more accurate methods to diagnose and treat Lyme disease and its' coinfections so that others will not be affected by the lifelong damage that tiny little tick can cause.

Finally, thank you to Dawn for her presence, resources and support. She is providing a support there for Wired Sisters everywhere, whether they are newly wired or on their third or fourth device. None of this is routine and having her there to connect all of us is so valuable and such a blessing.

Diane

I was not born with a heart condition. Being adopted, I don't know if I had any genetics for heart disease. But I have a serious heart issue. I found out the hard way that alcohol can negatively affect your heart.

I can count on one hand the number of drinks I had up until my 21st birthday – both of them at an after-performance celebration of a college theater production. Alcohol was not often found in my home; my parents did not have pre-dinner cocktails, nor did they have friends over for cocktails more than maybe once or twice a year. Thus I was not exposed to the temptation of alcohol at home. At college, the friends I hung out with were not drinkers either, so I don't remember us drinking at all. After college, I was living at home but working at large company with a very active employee organization. I got involved in their athletic teams – including softball, bowling, golf, and skiing. It is also where I became involved in social drinking. After every softball game, you could find us at a local restaurant with pitchers of beer. We had beer frames during bowling. Along with the bag of clubs, there was usually a six pack of beer in the golf cart. Skiing ended in front of the fireplace with wine and cheese. Since I worked at this company for almost 15 years, this became a way of life. Another member of this group was the great guy who would eventually become my husband.

After we married and bought our first house, we had frequent parties. People would come and bring a bottle or whatever – and because they left behind what they had not drunk, we always had a supply of liquor in the house. My self-control was tested, and often lost.

Fast forward to 2007. By this time I was drinking regularly, as in daily. I also had become pretty sedentary, no longer participating in team sports, or sports of any type for that matter. I went to work, came home and had a few drinks while making dinner, ate dinner, and then either sat in front of the television or in front of the computer, frequently with a snack in front of me. So it is no surprise my weight was going up, up and up (peaking at almost 210), while my energy level and activity were going down, down, and down. There was always a nagging thought in my mind that what I was doing wasn't good for me, but I pushed it aside. My friends and family expressed concern. But in my mind, if I didn't acknowledge it, it wouldn't be true.

By late 2007, my weight was up (over 200 pounds) and my energy level was pretty low. I was experiencing shortness of breath whenever I walked – which I attributed to being overweight. On December 7th, I was so short of breath when walking that my husband convinced me I needed to go to the hospital. And he really had to work at convincing me. Eventually I went – but only after having a few drinks to boost my confidence. His persistence may well have saved my life.

First eye-opener. When the triage nurse put the device on my finger to measure my pulse, she thought it was broken because she couldn't get a reading. She did a manual reading and realized my pulse was over 205 beats per minute. Next was an EKG. Then there was a flurry of activity in my room. The ER doctor was telling me I was in serious condition. One nurse was putting in an IV; another was inserting a Foley catheter. I had a blood pressure cuff on my arm taking a reading every couple of minutes. There were machines beeping. I had been in the ER before for stitches, but never for anything serious.

But I was still somewhat under the influence of the drinks I had tossed down before I went to the hospital so wasn't too concerned. I was admitted for tests. After what seemed like endless tests over the next couple of days, a cardiologist came to talk to me. He explained that the alcohol had negatively affected my heart. I would need to take medication, including Coumadin, for the rest of my life. I would need to exercise. I would need to watch my diet. Then he said something that really got my attention – "If you take another drink, you will die." Wow, brutally honest. But it got through to me.

I had a serious medical problem and it was my fault – I had done this to myself. That first visit I was in the hospital for 17 days for testing and while they got my heart rate under control and tried various medications to find the ones that worked best. But I walked out of that hospital "on the wagon" and was determined to stay there.

The next year was very rough for me emotionally. My husband developed a severe medical condition, a version of Lou Gehrig's disease. His leg muscles were deteriorating. He was no longer able to work and had to give up golf. But he inspired me by facing his fight with courage. He knew there was no cure for what he had and it was only going to get worse. I told myself that if he could do that, I could face not having alcohol in my life. But it was rough. I hadn't realized the extent to which I relied on alcohol to help me face problems.

In September 2008, my husband fell down the basement stairs and broke his neck. He lost consciousness immediately and never regained it. On the surface, I was relieved for his sake because he was no longer in pain and would not have to deal anymore with the dread of what the future was going to bring. Deep inside I was devastated. The temptation to turn back to alcohol was so very strong – but I am proud to say I didn't do it.

I thought my heart problem was under control. I was taking Coumadin and getting my INR tested regularly. I was taking other heart medications as well. I felt pretty good with only occasional bouts of loss of energy. I was still overweight, but I knew it was because I was just not eating correctly.

Then at work one day, I remember thinking I had just put my head down on my desk for a moment to rest. But one of my co-workers was concerned because I was very pale and shaky.

My boss called my cardiologist; he thought it may have been due to a low sugar level or something and didn't seem to be too concerned. But my coworkers felt otherwise and convinced me to let them call an ambulance. The fire station was literally across the street from my office and the paramedics were there in less than 5 minutes. Long story short – I arrested in the ambulance in the parking lot before we even left for the hospital and the paramedics brought me back. But I wasn't really aware of what was going on – they had given me something to relax me before they used the defibrillator. I woke up in the ER at a different hospital than I had been at previously. I was now seeing different doctors and had started on a different journey.

A cardiologist came in and told me the next day they were going to do an angiogram to see if I needed stents. As it turned out, I needed two of them. Then a doctor came in and introduced himself as an electrophysiologist. I had never heard the term before. But I wasn't concerned – until he told me I may need to have an ICD implanted. I was familiar with pacemakers, but had never heard of an ICD. When he explained why I needed it – that I had heart arrhythmia that could cause me to go into cardiac arrest again – I was scared. But I knew this was something I needed to have done.

Thus started my wired journey. Over the past four years, I have gone through numerous medications. One worked well at keeping the arrhythmia under control, but was negatively affecting other body organs so they took me off it.

I have had several cardioversions to deal with recurring afib. A few weeks ago I had an ablation for afib; it will take a few months to know if it has "cured" the afib but at my two week follow-up visit the results were promising. Over the four years, my ICD has delivered therapy several times. After the first one, which caught me totally by surprise, they didn't bother me – I have a mindset that of thankfulness for the device because it had saved my life again. What bothered me was the fact that after each time I received therapy, I was not allowed to drive for 6 months. Living in the suburbs where there is really no public transportation and nothing is within walking distance, this at first was an issue I thought was bigger than it turned out to be. When my last two therapies were delivered only 6 months and 1 week apart, I realized that six months is really no magic number. Just because I pass the six month mark doesn't mean I won't have therapy delivered again. I now accept that I will never drive again. I won't endanger anyone else by passing out behind the wheel. But I am dealing with it, thanks to friends and family who make sure I get to church, to the store, to my doctors' appointments, etc. I frequently use taxis.

A bigger concern now is that there are no more medications for the doctors to try. I am on the last one and if I have another cardiac episode, it is likely that they will have to do an ablation to try to eliminate the VT that is causing the episodes. I understand that could be a risky procedure, so am hoping it doesn't become necessary. But if it does, I have complete confidence in my doctor and will have it done.

There is a reason I'm sharing my story – a moral, so to speak. I knew alcohol could cause liver disease. I knew it could cause weight gain. I knew driving under its influence could be deadly. But I never knew what it could do to your heart. I never knew it could damage the heart and cause cardiac arrest. I now have a dual identity. I am a recovering alcoholic. But I am also a heart patient with a serious problem that has serious consequences. If people ask me why I'm not drinking, and they do, I tell them honestly about how it affected my heart and how it is continuing to affect my life even though I haven't had a drink in years. It could have been avoided – had I only known then what I know now!

I am an active volunteer with a local organization that flies veterans to Washington DC. Through them, I was lucky to meet a cardiac nurse who specializes in EP. She was my rock in the beginning when I didn't know what questions to ask, etc. She is actually the one who introduced me to Wired4Life and I am so glad she did. While it is great to have her guidance, it isn't quite the same as hearing from people who are also going through the same thing. There are times when you just need to talk to a kindred soul who has been through the same battle and knows where your head is at.

The Wired4Life sisters have been wonderful – I love the camaraderie and exchanges of ideas. I can't wait for the conference next year where I will be able to meet the wonderful sisters I have had the opportunity to chat with and follow online.

Wired4Life has given me a new perspective on my wired situation. I am no longer scared of the unknown future because I know that I've either seen how my wired sisters have dealt with the same situation or else they will be there to give me advice and support.

Fran

The first time I remember having palpitations was in my teens. I think it was around 1993 when I was about 16. I was walking to the bus stop from college with friends. I had this really odd irregular thumping in my chest, I stopped walking for a bit until it passed and after a bit, forgot all about it.

After a while, palpitations became a common feature of my life, as did dizziness and shortness of breath when climbing stairs etc. I ignored it for quite a while, several years, hoping it would disappear of its own accord.

It wasn't until I went to University at age 19 that the symptoms cranked up a gear and the palpitations were starting to make me feel very unwell and for large parts of the day. I saw my GP who sent me to have a 24hr ECG Holter Monitor (I remember in those days the monitors were cassette personal stereo sized and quite chunky and heavy!). Less than 24hrs after returning the monitor I received a phone call asking me to come up to the hospital that afternoon. As you can imagine, kind of scary.

I met one of the general medical consultants who asked me a lot about my family history and my own (then quite small) medical history and told me I had something called SVT (supra-ventricular tachycardia) which is an abnormal heart rhythm originating in the top part of the heart.

He referred me to a cardiologist who suggested I have an EP Study (cardiac electrophysiology study, where thin flexible tubes called catheters are put into a vein, threaded up into the heart and the electrical system of the heart is tested from inside). He said that once they found the 'spot' generating the abnormal rhythm they could do an ablation (burn) to cure me. A cure! So of course I agreed.

The EP Study did not find SVT. They could not induce any abnormal rhythms at all, so I was discharged on heart medications.

For the next several years I saw cardiologist after cardiologist who told me that when my heart rate was fast, the rhythm was normal, so I must have an anxiety disorder. I was repeatedly dismissed. It drained me so much over the years that I stopped going to the doctors about it, unless I was very unwell with it. Many times I found myself in A&E (ER) due to very fast heart rates, but again was eventually sent home with no extra help because I was in "Sinus Tachycardia" (which is a normal heart rhythm). I fainted a number of times and was given an implanted heart monitor called a Reveal Device (very tiny little implant).

In the years that passed I became fascinated with cardiology. I had always loved biology and human biology in particular since I was a small child (I used to read my mum's biology text books in break at primary school!).

I had finished my Art Degree at University and found I really wanted to move into a medical field. I initially trained as a nurse, but part way through I decided I wanted to work specifically in cardiology, so got a post as a Student Cardiac Technician at a large teaching Hospital.

As I trained and learned my profession, I discovered that what was wrong with me was a condition called IST (Inappropriate Sinus Tachycardia). I was not anxious (which requires completely different treatment!); there was something physical going on. Fortunately, one Cardiologist I worked with who was an EP (Electrophysiologist) referred me to one of his colleagues who had a great deal of experience with complex ablations. I liked him immediately and I have been seeing him now for well in excess of 10 years.

This time, the EP Study and ablation was a great success, the area generating the IST was found and treated and they also found I had an arrhythmia called Atrial Flutter which they treated as well. My relief was immense! I had had a consistently high heart rate for years, the slightest exertion wore me out so quickly and now there was a chance that was all gone!

Unfortunately, within a few weeks I began to be very dizzy and tripped over a few times, I managed to injure my leg one time, so was given another 24hr ECG monitor.

The results showed I was having bradycardia (slow heart rate) down to around 35bpm (anything below 50 or 60 bpm is low depending on your level of fitness). I was also having 'pauses' where my heart would stop for 6 or 7 seconds at a time. My consultant offered me a pacemaker as I had managed to injure myself when I was dizzy.

I had very mixed feelings about getting a pacemaker. On the one hand, from looking after patients who had pacemakers, I could see that they dramatically improved people's quality of life. But I also knew, that at the age of 28, it meant a lifetime of 'box changes' (battery/pacemaker replacement) every 8 – 10 years or so. My colleagues joked with me about it being very funny to be receiving a pacemaker, given my job! One said "ah, just like a cardiologist needing a bypass!"

I had rather a bad time of it during the operation to put in the pacemaker. I'm sad to say that the operating doctor (who was not my specialist), did not really listen to me when I insisted I needed more local anesthetic and pain killers. I am thankful that the scrub nurse listened to me though and insisted the doctor address my pain eventually! I felt really shaken up by the experience. Not something I was expecting at all. I had heard most patients I'd previously spoken to say that having the pacemaker implanted was 'not too bad' an experience, some had had problems, but not most.

I felt dramatically better after getting the pacemaker! I only needed one lead (wire) into my Right Atrium (top, right chamber of the heart) as the AV junction between the top and bottom of my heart functioned perfectly. My energy levels improved so much! My specialist said that after they had ablated my IST, it turned out they found my Sinus Node (where the heart beat normally originates from) had been damaged over the years, possibly by the IST and was not able to function well enough all the time without help.

I did develop more arrhythmias over time, a very fast one called AVNRT with a rate of 275bpm! Also Atrial Fibrillation and some others. I had an ablation for the AVNRT, but have medication to control other arrhythmias now.

Pretty soon after having the pacemaker implanted I started to become very ill with many different symptoms, after a long diagnostic process, I was eventually diagnosed with Behçet's Disease. My Cardiologist suggested this may have been the cause of my heart problems. I won't go into how the Behçet's affected me in general, but needless to say that combined with the heart problems, my husband and I had several turbulent years with my health and him having to give up work to care for me. I also had to give up work as a cardiac technician, something I loved dearly and was good at.

Unfortunately, I developed Neuro-Behçet's and was seriously ill. My neurologist wanted me to have MRI scans which was impossible with my pacemaker and it wasn't until many years later that I learned of the development of MRI-Conditional Pacemakers that can allow an MRI scan to be performed safely. I knew from my previous profession that these devices were very new and I wanted to wait a bit until the technology was 'proven' in clinical practice. I waited 3 years, until I could not wait any longer. The Neuro-Behçet's was wreaking havoc and MRI scans would bring real benefit.

I had an MRI-Conditional Pacemaker in November 2013. This meant I had to have the old pacemaker removed and the old lead (wire) extracted under GA (general anesthesia). Even though I had worked in hospitals for many years and had been in as a patient many times too, I found myself very scared when I was taken into theatre. I remember shivering in my hospital gown and sitting on the edge of the table. The staff were all lovely though and took care of me so well. They recognized immediately how scared I was and helped me through it. The anesthesiologist in particular was very cheery with me. I appreciated that.

I had an awful time afterwards, perhaps I reacted badly to the GA. No-one is exactly sure, but the staff were worried that I'd had a stroke and sent me for a brain scan.

I was able to write down for them that the symptoms were probably due to my Behçet's, which is most likely and I recovered a few hours later. This was several hours of worry for my husband who, at 8pm had his first news of how I was since I went to theatre at 2pm!

After about 6 weeks of my heart being 'irritable' from having been poked and prodded – things calmed down and are generally ok. The experience felt traumatic again, in a different way from the first time, I'm glad it's over.

At this point, I'm awaiting my first MRI scan in over 10 years! Oddly I remember quite liking the sounds the machine makes (which I know most people do not). I think I'm just really grateful to so many people, that I'm still here, in one piece and am supported by amazing technology and technique, along with many highly skilled professionals who look after me so well.

If you are due to have a pacemaker or other implanted device and are a woman there are a few pieces of advice I would give to you:

- If your cardiologist does not talk to you about where your pacemaker is going to be implanted in your chest – then bring it up! I did not mind that my scar would be visible, but some people do and there are ways of implanting them so that the scars are hidden lower down.
- Buy a really supportive bra for after your surgery, you will need it! Especially if you are not small-chested.

- Get hold of a shoulder pad or another small fabric pad, you'll need this to put under your bra strap over the top of the scar/pacemaker whilst it heals (this applies if you have the pacemaker implanted in the 'traditional' place, which is under your bra strap on the left or sometimes, right).
- Make sure you have help in place for after the op. You won't be able to lift anything with the arm on the side that the pacemaker was implanted for a few weeks or raise that arm above your head. You might need help with shopping and washing and dressing, depending on how mobile you normally are.

I wish you all the best, my life has been made so much better for being wired, both physically and mentally.

Nelly

My name is Nelly I am 40 years old, I live in British Columbia, Canada. Some of my hobbies and interests include spending time with my two daughters; Kaylie 12 and Gabriella 11, they are wonderful children. Some of the things that the three of us enjoy doing include; hiking, bike rides, games, cooking, baking, all sorts of girly things; except shopping, I hate shopping!!!!!

Kaylie has a cat that sleeps with her every night and follows her all around the house when she's at school; she will lie on her bed till she comes home.

Gabriella has a puppy, hamster, bunny and two cats; she would take all stray animals home if I let her. Both girls do terrific in school, and I volunteer at the school to stay involved with their schooling. I work full time as a nurse currently in Geriatrics and palliative care.

Prior to my initial pacemaker implant I had no energy was frequently light-headed, many pre-syncopal as well as syncope spells, my heart rate would frequently be 30 at work and 20 at rest. I went to my GP many times, who said I was too young for cardiac problems!! I changed GP's insisted on the cardiac work up. The Holter monitor indicated a heart rate of 19 during the night and 25 at work at times!

I collapsed at work with a heart rate of 9 BPM, and was rushed to the ICU. Lines were put in; the crash cart was my best friend that day. I thank God this all happened at work and not at home.
I was diagnosed with Sick Sinus Syndrome and paced with a dual chamber cardiac pacemaker and most of my symptoms disappeared.

Prior to the initial implant I was scared; but also relieved that I finally got diagnosed, so I could go back to a normal lifestyle with energy for the girls and myself.

I just recently had my second pacemaker, I did well. Being on Coumadin created some challenges; they had to give me plasma and I ended up in the cardiac critical care cardiac unit for 8 days on heparin till my blood was at therapeutic level! I also had cardiac ablation done and the rate is in sinus rhythm now, this pacemaker should last 4 years.

At the time of next implant, I will also receive an additional lead placed alongside the existing one as one of the current leads is not functioning to its full capacity.

With my initial pacemaker implant I was looking for people with similar experiences and found the WIRED4LIFE support group! When I joined the group, it consisted of just a few members, now it has grown to larger numbers of women from all over the world, and I think that is absolutely fantastic. The support and education provided is awesome!

Dawn: I truly admire you; you've been a good friend and a great sister! Dawn has spent endless hours, energy and dedication to this support group, she's the glue that holds the W4L support group together.

To new members who are looking for support; you have found the right place! Within this group there are many ladies that have had similar experiences regarding issues surrounding the pacemaker and life's experiences! If you are going through a hard time and are comfortable sharing, the support will always be there. The members of this group provide emotional, spiritual and psychological support and experience.

Una

Hi, wired sisters, my name is Una and I'd like share my story with you! I was born on April 15, 1961 in a small country town in northwestern Minnesota. My parents told me that when I was three that doctors had discovered I had a heart murmur and that I would need surgery if the hole didn't close up. The decision was made to wait a few years, in the hope it would close on its own.

On July 3, 1968, when I was seven, I underwent open heart surgery for atrioventricular septal defect with a cleft in the mitral valve at the University of Minnesota Variety Children's Hospital. During the surgery, which lasted several hours, doctors discovered I had developed a complete heart block. The doctors figured the heart block would clear up on its own. I was hooked up to an external pacemaker,

During my hospital stay, I developed chorea, a nervous disease otherwise known as St. Vitus Dance. I was shaking the whole time. I also had pneumonia at the same time, this lasted several weeks.

I remember that my doctors were surprised I recovered as quickly as I did. My mom and dad told me this was because we had many, many people praying for us, but the doctors were skeptical.

They then told me I would need an implanted pacemaker to keep my heart beating normally. Without it, my heart would pace at only 42 beats a minute.

Doctors then implanted an internal mercury battery pacemaker the size of a large cigarette pack in my abdomen on August 5, 1968.

I can't remember feeling any different after my surgery. I was treated differently though. I wanted to run around but my mom and dad kept telling me to slow down, not to do so much. They were scared and kept their eyes on me so that I wouldn't become too overly active. They were also afraid I would get endocarditis, an infection in the lining of my heart, or that I would suffer from chorea all over again.

I had to put up with a regular regimen of penicillin shots to prevent infection, and iron pills because of the low levels of iron in my blood. Early photographs of me show me as thin and pale.

My parents gradually let friends and neighbors know of my pacemaker and told my schoolteachers as I went into second grade. I was always at the front of the line whenever my class went somewhere, so that nobody would bump into me. They were scared that if I got pushed around that a wire might break or the pacemaker would malfunction. I was also picked on quite a bit by other kids because I was different.

I was overprotected when I was younger because I couldn't take part in physical education classes at all, so I had to play by myself when other kids were having Phy Ed. I think some of the kids didn't like that, so I was shunned by a few students.

I soon got used to counting my pulse several times a day. My parents did this for me in the beginning, and then taught me how to do it for myself. At first, we didn't know what to expect if my pulse became erratic before I was scheduled to have my pacemaker changed. This was before the days when doctors could check to see how long the battery would last. We knew a little about when the battery might wear down and I would have to have it replaced before this time. During my school years my pacemaker malfunctioned three times in a five year period.

The next few years progressed pretty normally. I graduated from high school in 1979 and went on to Bethel College in St. Paul, Minnesota for a year. In the fall of 1980 I started working at REM Roseau, a home for multi- handicapped children in Roseau, MN.

The fall of 1983 brought more changes. I started college at what was then called St. Paul Bible College. While there I met Michael, originally from London, England. Our paths were to cross often on the 129-acre campus. We would often arrive at the same movie or shopping mall; even attend the same church without planning it beforehand.

We started courting after he invited me to a nearby Pentecostal church. He wanted to see how a nice Minnesota girl would react to Charismatic worship! Soon our friendship blossomed and it wasn't long before we realized that we really cared for each other, and we became inseparable.

We became engaged in April, 1984 and were married at a little Baptist church surrounded by sugar beet fields in Eagle Point, Minnesota, on May 17, 1986. I graduated with a Family/Child Development degree in May 1988. Our first born, Megan, arrived five weeks early in August 1988. I was able to start using my degree right away!! Emma was born in November 1991. I was able to have them both naturally and was able to breastfeed them.

The next few years went by fast. I was a stay-at-home mom and absolutely loved it. My health stayed good. I had my pacemakers changed when needed. Everything seemed to be going fine.
A family crisis came at the end of December 2003 when my dad died of a sudden heart attack. It was a shock since he had never had heart problems. We spent the New Year in northwestern Minnesota with my mom and my two sisters and their families. My older sister is five years older than I am, is married and lives the closest to my Mom. My younger sister is married with two children and lives in North Pole, Alaska.

On November 22, 2004, crisis hit again. While watching TV, I had a cardiac arrest. I was rushed to the ICU at St. Francis Hospital in Shakopee, Minnesota. I was put in an induced coma to help me rest and recover. I was breathing with a ventilator and developed ARDS -- Adult Respiratory Distress Syndrome, which is "direr than pneumonia."

I was critically ill and my life was hanging in the balance. It was quite possible that I would have permanent damage to my heart and brain. Friends were coming to the hospital to say their goodbyes. People all over the world were praying for my family and me.

I went into V-Fib early Friday evening, Dec 3, as I had on the 22nd of November, and my heart stopped beating again. The doctor and nurses had to paddle me and do CPR. I also received epinephrine to get my heart beating again. The pacemaker again refused to kick in and they saw the same erratic rhythm they found two weeks before, for whatever reason they do not know.

The doctor told Michael that my brain, slightly-damaged liver, and my kidneys were still functioning and that I still had brain stem activity; they still did not know about higher-level thinking ability. The difficulty was with my lungs and that my heart kept arresting. My husband was told the more this happens, the more damage there is to the body. The doctor said this was quite a serious setback considering the slow and gradual process I was making, and that I was in worse shape after this than when I first entered the hospital nearly two weeks before. Dr. Clara Wu said there was still some hope because she had seen people with similar cases survive after months of treatment, but not with such underlying heart and lung issues.

The doctors reduced the sedation Christmas Day, 2004, and I became the hospital's Christmas miracle. I awoke just before New Year's not realizing I had missed the previous six weeks. I did know I was in the hospital and that I was sick. However, I couldn't remember what happened the day I was taken to the hospital. I do remember songs going through my mind. I've been told that different people came in and sang to me. These songs touched my heart and kept me going. At the same time people prayed for me and I know I felt the powerful effect of their prayers.

One of my favorite memories while sleeping was of a 4-year-old boy, Joey, who came to visit me. He came with his mom and asked to lie beside me on the bed. The nurse said it was okay. He lay by me and told me that he missed me at church and that his sister did too. This was a few days before I fully woke up from the coma. I was able to ask Joey when he visited me at a later date if this happened and he said yes. Joey's mom also told me of how he would think of me in the middle of the day and that he would insist that they had to pray for me at that point in time.

In January, 2005 I was transferred to another hospital to have my pacemaker replaced with a pacemaker/defibrillator (ICD). This is now my twelfth device. After that I was sent to rehab for a month and came home just before Valentine's 2005. I came home with a walker and on oxygen full time. I was able to stop using the walker a few months later.

On August 4, 2006 I had open-heart surgery to replace a valve. Since then I have been able to come off oxygen completely. I am now back to where I was before I had my cardiac arrest. I've been told that I am better than ever. All this is because we have a wonderful, faithful, caring God. He hears our prayers and is there for us in all things.

My life verse is Psalm 73:25-26. It says: "Who have I in heaven but you? And besides You, I desire nothing on earth. My flesh and my heart may fail, but God is the strength of my heart and my portion forever,"

I live with my family in Chaska, MN, a suburb of Minneapolis/St. Paul. My oldest daughter is in her first year of college and our youngest is in tenth grade. My husband is a writer for ASSIST News Service, Christian wire service/news agency providing news and feature stories to media outlets across America and around the world.

I am a full time homemaker and love every moment of it. I help to take care of babies every other week for the Mothers of Preschool program at my church. My younger daughter and I also take care of babies every other Saturday night at church so parents can go out on a date. Besides taking care of babies, I like to read, do counted cross-stitch, and bake. I am a self-taught computer problem solver. I enjoy fixing things on our computers and keeping them maintained.

Mary Ellen

Several weeks ago Dawn and I exchanged some emails about the emotions I had after the pacemaker implanted. On June 16th 2012, it will be 2 ½ years since my Toy (what I call my pacemaker) was implanted in a chilly, crisp but sunny December morning, the Blessed month of the Christ Child's birth.

There are so many things I want to write about, tears, would I wake up in the mornings, will the scar be horrible, (I love low cut blouses) could I pack that 50 pound bag of feed? So many ups and downs.

I knew a couple of guys with pacemakers, and one is rather fragile. Men have heart problems, not women! About 3 or 4 months after the implant I learned about Dawn and WIRED4LIFE, a dear friend found an article in Heart Healthy magazine. I visited with Dawn on the phone for a long time, goodness how I kept her on that phone, but she was so helpful and patient, soothing my nerves. I was happy to know I was not the only woman with a pacemaker! I had never met a woman with a pacemaker!

Thinking back when I started fainting, a total of 7 times, once in the hospital, once in the doctor's office, another time I got out of bed walked to the bathroom started to brush my teeth and fainted!

I was so very tired all the time, so weak. I would hand wash the dishes and I got tired. I remember once we went to a classic car show and I did not have the energy to get out of a folding chair, Benny that had to help me, literally pulling me up. To climb the stairs at home was slow process and I would be exhausted at the top. I was light headed, my legs weak and sort of tingled. I even worried had I gained a lot of weight, but all my clothes still fit.

Every Wednesday we meet for breakfast with our car club, friends would tell me I looked pale, my hands were colorless and I was just plain tired. I almost felt like I had become useless, not happy about anything, just could not get motivated.

One afternoon, trying to stay busy I stopped at an antique shop, I found this wonderful very old and yellowed (1895), framed print, it read, "What time I am afraid, I will trust in Thee."

After the angiogram, and heart monitoring tests. The Dr. Whitehill, EP Cardiologist tells me I need a pacemaker. I tried not to cry in his office, but when Benny and I got in the pickup, I screamed and cried until I was worn out. Heavenly Father and all the Saints be with me, I so scared, I saw tears in my love one's eyes and I cried, big never ending tears, just when I thought I had ran out of tears, they start all over again.

I cried and remembered all my family that now lives in Heaven, my son, my parents, I remember holding onto the railing on the hospital bed so tight.

Yes, ladies there were times I was so worried I would not see, my one and only darling granddaughter grow up, perhaps married and having her own babies. What priceless treasure and memory that would for me.

How very frightened I was when I was wheeled into that very menacing operating room, at least to me it was the most menacing place in the world. Would I be wheeled out alive? Would I become disabled in a wheelchair? I didn't want this pacemaker, but here I was being wheeled into that room at about 7:30 am. I was never put to sleep. Back in my room by 9:00, walking the hallway by 10, breakfast/lunch about 11 and home by 12 noon! And guess what the scar is very fine, done vertical instead of horizontal. Silly me worrying about a scar.

Suddenly I had this St. Jude's pacemaker and Praise the Lord, I felt wonderful, sore as heck, but I could see pink in my hands, my face. I remember feeling so happy, ready to face Christmas and the rest of my life, cooking like it was going out of style! Benny was so wonderful, so helpful, even cutting the meat for me, reminding me to be careful, don't lift the arm up high, don't carry that, I'll do it. He even drives me to get a pedicure, grocery store or where ever. He is afraid I will faint while driving.

But then came the day I was frightened again, how long would this pacemaker last? Anxiety/insecurity like a depression took hold of me, I endured upset stomachs, crying for no reason? I would lay in bed listening to my heart. If I did any activity my heart would start racing, not realizing that was good. I knew Benny needed his wife, but I was afraid of intimacy. I would look at that antique print, I'm trying heavenly Father, but it's so hard!

Think I called Dawn or perhaps just emailed several times with questions, she would sometimes say check with your doctor, and this is not related to the pacemaker.

The nurses helped, but I was not getting all the answers I needed. My health had improved, my energy was up to speed. Every time I visit the technician, all was well. My cardiologist was happy with all re-ports, my family doctor ordered blood work, no diabetes, and no cholesterol, a little low on potassium, my blood pressure is running about 140 over 80 and at almost 72 years old, I have a new lease at life.

My cardiologist now wants to see me about once a year and the technician every 6 months. Still I had a few concerns. I walk around our acres and I have used a stair master up to 30 minutes every day. My left arm is not as strong as I would like it to be, the armpit has a strange tug when I try to lift something over my head that has to do with the pacemaker.

One morning in desperation I called St. Jude Medical, God bless that young man on the phone, and he had the patience of Job, with my 20 plus questions, slowly and carefully explaining everything. I told him I lived about 40 miles from the doctor's office, hey, what happens when the battery runs out, he says hang on, you can listen to the sound, my pacemaker sounds like a British ambulance. I had to laugh, I had visions of myself at church, a car show or some store, running into someone, giving them a big Texas hug and the ambulance goes off.

I was assured I had about 30 days of battery life left, so call the doctor office right away. The one thing I have definitely learned in these 2 ½ years, the world is not going to stop because I did not clean my house. If my Benny wants me to go to the car parts store, I go. I no longer save the extra nice clothes for that special day, every day is special I wear those clothes with high heels and I wear my makeup daily!

There is no such thing as half-empty glass, it is half full and if it's a little sour I make cornbread! Now I sleep well, no problem, either side, I sleep peacefully. I thank God for every day, even when I stub my toe! "Lord I know this day is good."

I sincerely want with all my heart say thank you to all these ladies that have written their stories, I read and re-read all the stories. With some of your stories I cried for and with you and have prayed for your healing.

I'm sure that some of you cannot imagine how you helped me in accepting my pacemaker and realizing I had many years left of life, and only God can make that choice, God had given these heart doctors the ability and learning to perform this miracle for us. God, his Angels and all the Saints bless all those wonderful doctors. And God send blessings to Dawn and WIRED4LIFE group. In God's Peace and trust in him, with Texas hugs to all, Mary Ellen

WIRED SISTER VISITS

A treat for me personally was when a wired sister would be passing through Minneapolis-St. Paul, perhaps on her way somewhere else or specifically to visit me. The first non-local sister was Barbe', in Minneapolis for a work conference, from Alaska! We met for dinner and proceeded to talk well past the dinner hour; we have remained steadfast friends.

Wired "Auntie" Sherry from Kentucky specifically came to visit me, which was such a treat! I had been 'adopted' by many of the wired women in our group; I was a niece, sister, even daughter.

For our own family vacations, we set our sights on road trips that would bring me closer to my wired sisters. A visit to Hershey, Pennsylvania resulted in meeting my wired mom Jane, for the very first time. A few years later a trip to Maine to see Jean-Marie and Joyce, who lived in the same town and also met each other for the first time.

FACEBOOK

Facebook has been a life changer for our group. *In April 2016, we made the decision that we would be exclusively on Facebook with two separate pages and one private group.*

WIRED4LIFE for all; wired or not, friends, family who support people living with an implanted pacemaker, defibrillator, stent or heart valve. Providing education & information relating to their cardiac implants.

WIRED4LIFE Kids, which supports the parents of wired children or the wireds themselves!

PETS AND PACEMAKERS

1) Harlan and Nancy Weikle of For Paws Hospice and Red Flyer, The Handicapped Pet organization, became involved with WIRED4LIFE when Harlan called to inquire about finding a working pacemaker for a dog. It seems like such a small, enclosed world at times, and then these conversations turn into lifelong friendships.

2) "Buddy the Jack Russell with a Pacemaker" dog and owner Andrew Lefcourt are friends on Facebook!

(The following content is courtesy of Squidoo and JohannTheDog) In 1968, just eight years after the first human received a pacemaker, the first pup received one of these life saving devices in an historic surgery performed by James W. Buchanan at the School of Veterinary Medicine, University of Pennsylvania.

It is estimated that over 300-400 dogs receive pacemakers every year for applicable heart conditions, even though about 4000 dogs are in need.

There are no pacemakers made specifically for veterinary use. Devices used by veterinarians are either units with good battery life that have been donated by human patients following their death, or are units provided at no cost by manufacturing companies after the pacemakers' shelf expiration date has passed.

"Pacemakers in dogs correct the same abnormalities as they do in people," according to Alan Spier, assistant professor of veterinary cardiology, University of Missouri-Columbia (MU). "We receive many phone calls from people with pacemakers, or their family members, expressing desire to donate the pacemakers after the individual's death. Many people feel strongly that this is an important gesture."

WARM FUZZIES

Through the years I've received countless emails, letters in the mail, phone calls, texts, and e-cards from our wired sisters, sharing their gratitude and admiration for what I do. I've always called them "warm fuzzies," because to me, that is what they have accomplished. They are little reminders; words from the heart that encourage and give me the drive and determination to keep this mission going.

For the most part, WIRED4LIFE has been my baby. I've driven the bus, and heck – even learned to parallel park it. When I've needed help, it has come, and for that – I send warm fuzzies out. The world needs people who can make a difference, to move an immovable mountain, and oftentimes these gifts came in the form of money or services, a favor, paid for a class that needed to be taken, or advice that came from experience.

The power of the written word is mighty, and when woven in with gratitude, it can move those mountains.

I have been part of this group less than a week and I am already so impressed. I have not known you long, but your compassion and good sense shines through cyberspace.

Dawn, you know how grateful I've been for all you do for your wired sisters. This is just one more thing above and beyond the call. Thank you so much!

I'm glad you have had such success with your support group. It's amazing how little people know about pacers when they get them; how little they are informed of what to expect; and how so very helpful it is to have support groups - especially when things do not go by the textbook. Keep up the good work!

Once again, you have created a wonderful newsletter for all of us to enjoy! You are just incredible and I thank God for your leadership in our wonderful group of ladies.

Just wanted to tell you how much I enjoyed the newsletter. As usual, you have done a perfect job and all of us should thank you from the bottom of our hearts.

Great newsletter. Learn something new each time. Never heard of a "heart stunning" event related to stress. Forwarded to a few stressed out gal friends. Thanks for all your creativity and work.

Thanks Dawn....that is interesting newsletter....so glad to be part of the group!

Thanks for everything you do for the group, I really do appreciate the newsletter each time it arrives in my inbox!

I love the new format, very interesting and fun to read, you put a lot of effort into it! Thank you very much Dawn for everything. God Bless you for putting this group together.

I finished reading the newsletter. Beautiful job. I enjoyed reading all of it. I liked the section on Ablation. I didn't know what it was before. The pictures were great. Looking forward to next month's newsletter.

You do a fabulous job on the newsletters and I read them from cover to cover………You do a lot of work for all of us and I hope that everyone appreciates you……..

We have a spiritual bond that grows stronger each year.
We're not sisters by birth but we've known from the start.
God put us together to be Sisters by Heart

If I had a million years it wouldn't be long enough to tell you how thrilled I am to have found this group! Thank you so much for providing such a wonderful place for 'wired' women to go. I always thought that my first implant date was one of the most important dates in my life, now I've added finding your WIRED4LIFE group to my list of treasured dates. My heart is truly touched.

….I became a member. It was great to have other women who deal with issues related to pacemakers, to chat, share, vent or just cry with. I am already making my vacation plans to attend the conference

I found WIRED4LIFE by accident, while looking for support groups, as I had questions about the size of my pacemaker and some of the feelings that came with it. I am thrilled with the group, the kindness of Dawn and of the others who have welcomed me to the group.

I have found that there are a LOT of groups out there, for all ages and with all kinds of problems, but it's especially nice to have a website just for women.

WIRED CONFERENCES

A frequent conversation-getter in our Saturday morning chats was that the women wanted to meet. In person, at one time. Having a very diverse career background which included the necessary skills to make this happen (extraordinary organization, travel and event planning and knowing how to ask for what you need), it was a task I jumped on. We were based in the Twin Cities at the time, as were the top three device manufacturers; Boston Scientific, St. Jude Medical and Medtronic. Imagine!

Perhaps a few days to learn about our devices and some 'girly' stuff (shopping, munching on chocolate, spending quality time together) - what could be better? Indeed.

Our first Gathering was in 2009, and they have continued every "odd" year through 2015. We also have mini-gatherings for our local sisters; this might include lunch out and/or a visit to a device maker!
We are very thankful to Boston Scientific and Medtronic for rolling out the red carpet for our group. Tours, goodie bags, lunch and most importantly, the opportunity to share our stories with the people that make it possible for us to do so. Time together with wired sisters; is a perfect prescription for good heart health!

MISSION STATEMENT

We support our wired community by providing education, emotional support and friendship.

GUEST CONTRIBUTORS

Aside from wired sisters sharing their stories, and our cardiac nurse/wired sister Jill maintaining her "Ask a Nurse" column, we have had frequent contributors to the newsletter. Some had their own columns which might relate to the monthly theme of the newsletter, or for the time or season of year. Dixie's column was titled "Heart to Heart," she shared with us life in her own neighborhood, focusing on issues relating directly to women, tips on recovery from surgery, living healthy and happy.

Lynette Crane, a Certified Life Coach and friend to WIRED, shared her own story with heart disease, although not 'wired' she was humbled by a heart attack and in turn was able to use her own story to educate and support busy women.

On occasion, wired sister Tammy would engage us with her 'ramblings' (her words) in "Tammy's Corner." Tammy had the innate ability to take a stubborn or difficult situation and turn it into a learning tool for us. From the July 2011 issue: "Having a pacemaker makes you as exotic as a two-headed purple parrot that can speak French." Her focus with that statement was that 'we are rare.' We are not necessarily 92 years old, we are oftentimes between the ages of 30-49 and living wired has been considered by some as we are 'fragile or broken.'

Tina inspired with very healthy recipes, and thoughts relating to spirit and grace, wisdom and reflection.

DEVICE MANUFACTURERS

Our relationships with the device manufacturers have remained strong. I am deeply indebted to them for their continuing work, research and development, patient education and support and their desire to give us a longer and healthier life to live.

There are other device manufacturers, but my experience has only been with Boston Scientific, Medtronic and St. Jude Medical. The information here has been provided by these specific companies and what is listed has been approved as content for this book.

Technology is changing so incredibly fast it can boggle the mind. To think that a pacemaker the size of a fingernail can be implanted into the heart without one wire attached is no longer a vision in the future, it is happening right now. The device manufacturers each have distinct cardiac device products. Please explore their websites for specific information. This information is listed below, as well as their mission statements!

Boston Scientific/Abbott

http://www.bostonscientific.com/en-US/health-conditions.html
Health conditions and products for patients with cardiac implants.

We are committed to transforming lives through innovative medical solutions that improve the health of patients around the world.

Medtronic

http://www.medtronic.com/patients/index.htm
Exploring options for your health conditions & living with an implanted cardiac device or therapy.

To contribute to human welfare by application of biomedical engineering in the research, design, manufacture, and sale of instruments or appliances that alleviate pain, restore health, and extend life.

St. Jude Medical

http://health.sjm.com
Common questions & answers, as well as specific product information, medical animations and patient videos.

We are driven by our vision and mission to transform the treatment of expensive epidemic diseases, including atrial fibrillation, heart failure, stroke, coronary artery disease, congenital heart defects, Parkinson's disease and chronic pain. St. Jude Medical is uniquely positioned to achieve our goal by providing innovative solutions that reduce the economic burden of costly diseases on health care systems worldwide and provide improved outcomes for patients.

ENCYLOPEDIA

This section will detail the primary indicators, procedures, tests and medical terminology that are appropriate for those with an implanted cardiac device; not all are listed here, but a vast majority are.

WHAT IS A PACEMAKER? ©2014, WebMD, LLC. All rights reserved

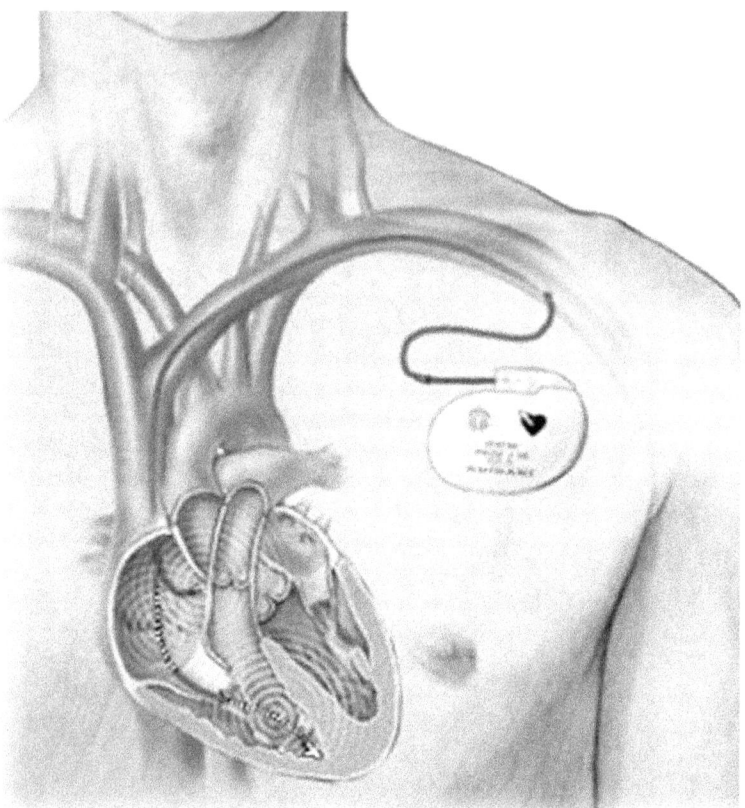

Your heartbeat is controlled by the heart's own bioelectrical triggering system. When that system ceases to work properly, the solution may be a pacemaker. A pacemaker is a small, battery-operated device that helps the heart beat in a regular rhythm. It is used to replace a faulty natural pacemaker or blocked pathway.

There are two types of pacemakers, permanent and temporary. Permanent pacemakers are called internal while the temporary type is called external.

- A pacemaker uses batteries to send electrical impulses to the heart to help it pump properly. An electrode is placed next to the heart wall and small electrical charges travel through the wire to the heart.
- Most pacemakers have a sensing device that turns itself off when the heartbeat is above a certain level. It turns back on when the heartbeat is too slow. These are called demand pacemakers.
- The pacemaker has two parts -- a battery-powered generator and the wires that connect it to the heart. The silver-dollar-size generator, which has an effective life of seven to 12 years, is implanted just beneath the skin below the collarbone. The leads are threaded into position through veins leading back to the heart.

Most patients with pacemakers suffer from a condition in which the heart beats too slowly (brady arrhythmia). This is most commonly a result of deterioration in the heart's own pacing system in elderly patients, though high blood pressure, coronary artery disease or scarring from a heart attack can also cause Brady arrhythmias.

The most commonly implanted pacing device is a demand pacemaker. It monitors the heart's activity and takes control only when the heart rate falls below a programmed minimum -- usually 60 beats per minute.

Other conditions which require pacemakers include heart block, in which the heart stops beating altogether for several seconds and tachyarrhythmia, an overly rapid heartbeat.

A more sophisticated type of pacemaker actually monitors a number of physical changes in the body, which signal an increase or decrease in activity. If the heart's own pacing system fails to respond properly, these rate-responsive pacemakers slowly raise or lower the heartbeat to the appropriate level from 60 to 150 beats per minute.

If the patient's condition dictates reprogramming the implanted generator, the cardiologist signals the changes to its tiny on-board computer with an electromagnetic signaling device placed on the surface of the skin above the pacemaker.

How does a pacemaker work?
The pacemaker essentially does two things: it senses the patient's own rhythm using a "sensing circuit", and it sends out electrical signals using an "output circuit". If the patient's intrinsic rhythm becomes too slow or goes away completely, the electronic pacemaker senses that, and starts sending out signals along the wires leading from the control box to the heart muscle. The signals, if they're "capturing" properly, provide a regular electrical stimulus, making the heart contract at a rate fast enough to maintain the patient's blood pressure.

What happens after the pacemaker is implanted?

Once the incision completely heals (which takes about 2 – 4 weeks,) the patient can largely return to a completely normal life. In fact, since pacemakers alleviate the symptoms of bradycardia, many patients find they are able to do even more after a pacemaker is implanted.

Periodic pacemaker checks are necessary, to measure the function of the device and the amount of energy left in the battery. The "scheduled maintenance" for pacemakers generally consists of periodic telephone follow-up (every month or two,) and usually yearly visits to the doctor's office. The telephone follow-up is a simple procedure consisting of placing a special "trans-telephonic follow-up device" over the pacemaker, and transmitting data over the telephone.

When the battery begins to get low, the doctor schedules an elective pacemaker replacement. This procedure is similar to the implantation procedure, except that usually the pacemaker leads do not need to be replaced. Under local anesthesia, the incision is opened, the generator is detached from the leads and thrown away, a new generator is attached, and the incision is then closed. (This is not merely a "battery change," though doctors sometimes call it that. No batteries are changed; instead, the entire old generator is discarded and a brand new one is placed.)

Life with a device

Following the suggested maintenance schedule usually means that pacemaker problems will be detected before they become serious. However, it is important for patients to be aware of the symptoms of bradycardia, symptoms that might indicate a pacemaker malfunction. Once again, these symptoms include weakness, easy fatigability, lightheadedness, dizziness, or loss of consciousness. Patients experiencing any of these symptoms should notify their doctor. A simple telephone check of the pacemaker is usually enough to rule out a pacemaker problem.

What are the parts of a pacemaker?

The pacemaker box itself is called the "pulse generator" – the generator is connected to either one or two wires, which carry the electrical signals to the heart muscle. Permanent pacing generators are implanted in the chest under the skin – nowadays they're very small – and the wires leading to the heart are threaded through the subclavian vein. The generator box consists of a small computerized chip controller that's run by a battery. The box senses and paces through the same set of wires that lead to the endocardium.

WHAT IS AN IMPLANTABLE CARDIOVERTER-DEBIFBRILLATOR (ICD)? ©2014, WebMD, LLC. All rights reserved

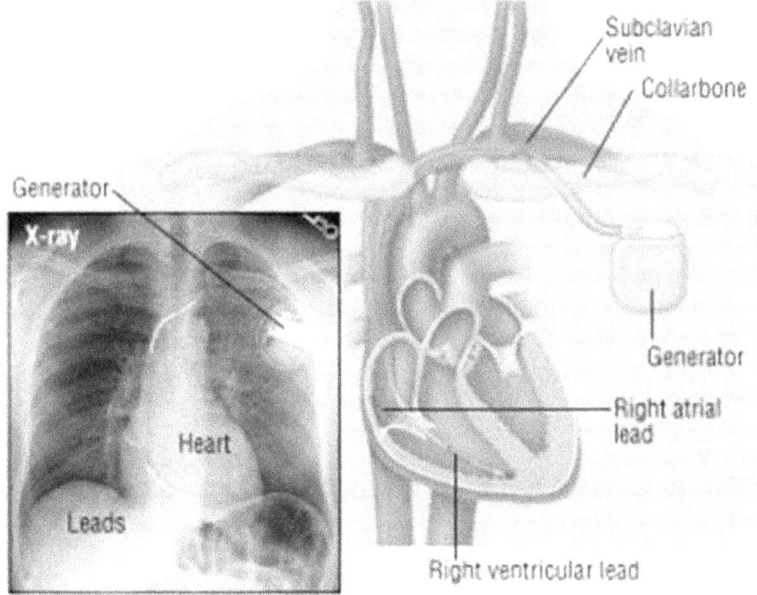

An implantable cardioverter-defibrillator (ICD) is a battery-powered device that can fix an abnormal heart rate or rhythm and prevent sudden death. The DEFIBRILLATOR is placed inside the chest. It's attached to one or two wires (called leads) that go into the heart through a vein. An ICD is also known as an automatic implantable cardioverter-defibrillator (AICD).

Who needs an ICD?
You might need an ICD if you have had a serious episode of an abnormally fast heart rhythm or are at high risk for having one. If you have coronary artery disease, heart failure, or a problem with the structure or electrical system of the heart, you may be at risk for an abnormal heart rhythm.

An example of a life-threatening heart rhythm is ventricular tachycardia.

How does an ICD work?
An ICD is always checking your heart rate and rhythm. If the ICD detects a life-threatening rapid heart rhythm, it tries to slow the rhythm to get it back to normal. If the dangerous rhythm does not stop, the ICD sends an electric shock to the heart to restore a normal rhythm. The device then goes back to its watchful mode.

An ICD also can fix a heart rate that is too fast or too slow. It does so without using a shock. It can send out electrical pulses to speed up a heart rate that is too slow. Or it can slow down a fast heart rate by matching the pace and bringing the heart rate back to normal.

Whether you get pulses or a shock depends on the type of problem that you have and how the doctor programs the ICD for you.

How is an ICD placed?
Your doctor will put the ICD in your chest during minor surgery. You will not have open-chest surgery. You probably will have local anesthesia. This means that you will be awake but feel no pain. You also will likely have medicine to make you feel relaxed and sleepy.

Your doctor makes a small cut (incision) in your upper chest. He or she puts one or two leads (wires) in a vein and threads them to the heart. Then your doctor connects the leads to the ICD. Your doctor programs the ICD and then puts it in your chest and closes the incision.

In some cases, the doctor may be able to put the ICD in another place in the chest so that you don't have a scar on your upper chest. This would allow you to wear clothing with a lower neckline and still keep the scar covered.

Most people spend the night in the hospital, just to make sure that the device is working and that there are no problems from the surgery. You may be able to see a little bump under the skin where the ICD is placed.

How does it feel to get a shock (or receive therapy) from an ICD?
The shock from an ICD hurts briefly. It's been described as feeling like a punch in the chest. But the shock is a sign that the ICD is doing its job to keep your heart beating. You won't feel any pain if the ICD uses electrical pulses to fix a heart rate that is too fast or too slow.

There's no way to know how often a shock might occur. It might never happen.

It's possible that the ICD could shock your heart when it shouldn't. You also might be afraid or worried about when the ICD might shock you again. But you can take simple steps to feel better about having an ICD. These include having your ICD checked regularly by your doctor and making an action plan for what to do if you get shocked.

How do I live a normal, healthy life with an ICD?

- Avoid strong magnetic and electrical fields. These can keep your device from working right. Most office equipment and home appliances are safe to use. Learn which things you should use with caution and which you should stay away from.
- Know what to do when you get a shock from your ICD.
- Be sure that any doctor, dentist, or other health professional you see knows that you have an ICD.
- Always carry a card in your wallet that tells what kind of device you have. Wear medical alert jewelry that says you have an ICD.
- Have your ICD checked regularly to make sure it's working right.
- It's common to be anxious that the ICD might shock you. But you can take steps to think positively and worry less about living with an ICD.

WHAT IS HEART VALVE DISEASE? ©2014, WebMD, LLC. All rights reserved

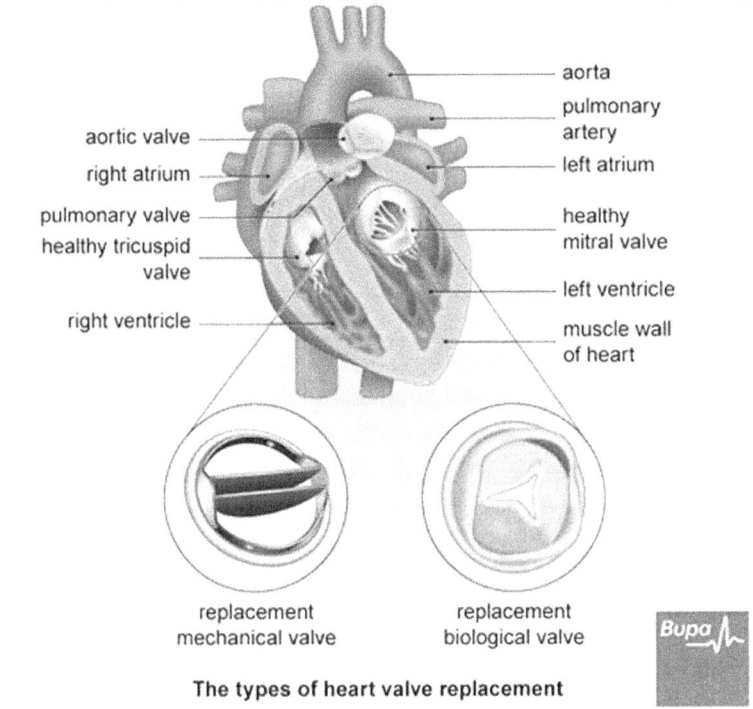

The types of heart valve replacement

Heart valve disease occurs when the heart valves do not work the way they should.

Your heart valves lie at the exit of each of your four heart chambers and maintain one-way blood flow through your heart. The four heart valves make sure that blood always flows freely in a forward direction and that there is no backward leakage.

Blood flows from your right and left atria into your ventricles through the open tricuspid and mitral valves.

When the ventricles are full, the tricuspid and mitral valves shut. This prevents blood from flowing backward into the atria while the ventricles contract.

As the ventricles begin to contract, the pulmonic and aortic valves are forced open and blood is pumped out of the ventricles. Blood from the right ventricle passes through the open pulmonic valve into the pulmonary artery, and blood from the left ventricle passes through the open aortic valve into the aorta and the rest of the body.

When the ventricles finish contracting and begin to relax, the aortic and pulmonic valves shut. These valves prevent blood from flowing back into the ventricles.

This pattern is repeated over and over with each heartbeat, causing blood to flow continuously to the heart, lungs, and body.

There are several types of heart valve disease:

- Valvular stenosis. This occurs when a heart valve doesn't fully open due to stiff or fused leaflets. The narrowed opening may make the heart work very hard to pump blood through it. This can lead to heart failure and other symptoms (see below). All four valves can develop stenosis; the conditions are called tricuspid stenosis, pulmonic stenosis, mitral stenosis, or aortic stenosis.

- Valvular insufficiency. Also called regurgitation, incompetence, or "leaky valve," this occurs when a valve does not close tightly. If the valves do not seal, some blood will leak backwards across the valve. As the leak worsens, the heart has to work harder to make up for the leaky valve, and less blood may flow to the rest of the body. Depending on which valve is affected, the condition is called tricuspid regurgitation, pulmonary regurgitation, mitral regurgitation, or aortic regurgitation.

What Causes Heart Valve Disease?
Heart valve disease can develop before birth (congenital) or can be acquired sometime during one's lifetime. Sometimes, the cause of valve disease is unknown.

- Congenital valve disease. This form of valve disease most often affects the aortic or pulmonic valve. Valves may be the wrong size, have malformed leaflets, or have leaflets that are not attached correctly.
- Bicuspid aortic valve disease is a congenital valve disease that affects the aortic valve. Instead of the normal three leaflets or cusps, the bicuspid aortic valve has only two. Without the third leaflet, the valve may be stiff (unable to open or close properly) or leaky (not able close tightly).
- Acquired valve disease. This includes problems that develop with valves that were once normal. These may involve changes in the structure or your valve due to a

variety of diseases or infections, including rheumatic fever or endocarditis.

- Rheumatic fever is caused by an untreated bacterial infection (usually strep throat). Luckily, this infection was much more common before the introduction of antibiotics to treat it in the 1950s. The initial infection usually occurs in children and causes inflammation of the heart valves. However, symptoms associated with the inflammation may not be seen until 20-40 years later.
- Endocarditis occurs when germs, especially bacteria, enter the bloodstream and attack the heart valves, causing growths and holes in the valves and scarring. This can lead to leaky valves. The germs that cause endocarditis can enter the blood during dental procedures, surgery, IV drug use, or with severe infections. People with valve disease can be at higher risk for developing endocarditis.

There are many changes that can occur to the valves of the heart. The chordae tendinae or papillary muscles can stretch or tear; the annulus of the valve can dilate (become wide); or the valve leaflets can become fibrotic (stiff) and calcified.

- Mitral valve prolapse (MVP) is a very common condition, affecting 1% to 2% of the population. MVP causes the leaflets of the mitral valve to flop back into the left atrium during the heart's contraction. MVP also causes the tissues of the valve to become abnormal and stretchy, causing the valve to leak. However, the condition rarely causes symptoms and usually doesn't require treatment.

Other causes of valve disease include: coronary artery disease, heart attack, cardiomyopathy (heart muscle disease), syphilis (a sexually transmitted disease), high blood pressure, aortic aneurysms, and connective tissue diseases. Less common causes of valve disease include tumors, some types of drugs, and radiation.

What Are the Symptoms of Heart Valve Disease?

- Shortness of breath and/or difficulty catching your breath. You may notice this most when you are active (doing your normal daily activities) or when you lie down flat in bed. You may need to sleep propped up on a few pillows to breathe easier.
- Weakness or dizziness. You may feel too weak to carry out your normal daily activities. Dizziness can also occur, and in some cases, passing out may be a symptom.
- Discomfort in your chest. You may feel a pressure or weight in your chest with activity or when going out in cold air.
- Palpitations. This may feel like a rapid heart rhythm, irregular heartbeat, skipped beats, or a flip-flop feeling in your chest.

- Swelling of your ankles, feet, or abdomen. This is called edema.
- Rapid weight gain. A weight gain of two or three pounds in one day is possible.

Symptoms of heart valve disease do not always relate to the seriousness of your condition. You may have no symptoms at all and have severe valve disease, requiring prompt treatment. Or, as with mitral valve prolapse, you may have noticeable symptoms, yet tests may show the valve leak is not significant.

How Are Heart Valve Diseases Diagnosed?
Your heart doctor can tell if you have heart valve disease by talking to you about symptoms, performing a physical exam, and performing other tests.

During a physical exam, the doctor will listen to your heart to hear sounds the heart makes as the valves open and close. A murmur is a swishing sound made by blood flowing through a stenotic or leaky valve. A doctor can also tell if the heart is enlarged or if your heart rhythm is irregular.

The doctor will listen to the lungs to hear if you are retaining fluid there, which shows the heart is not able to pump as well as it should.
By examining your body, the doctor can find clues about circulation and the functioning of other organs.

After the physical exam, the doctor may order diagnostic tests. These may include:

- Echocardiography
- Transesophageal echocardiography
- Cardiac catheterization (also called an angiogram)

By conducting some or all of these tests over time, your doctor can also see the progress of valve disease. This will help him or her make decisions about treatment.

How Is Heart Valve Disease Treated?

Heart valve disease treatment depends on the type and severity of disease. There are three goals of treatment for heart valve disease: protecting your valve from further damage; lessening symptoms; and repairing or replacing valves.

Aortic Valve Replacement Surgery

Aortic valve replacement is a surgery done for aortic valve stenosis and aortic valve regurgitation.
The surgery is either an open-heart surgery or a minimally invasive surgery. In an aortic valve replacement surgery, the damaged valve is removed and replaced with an artificial valve.

How is it done?

During open-heart valve surgery, the doctor makes a large incision in the chest. Blood is circulated outside of the body through a machine to add oxygen to it (cardiopulmonary bypass or heart-lung machine). The heart may be cooled to slow or stop the heartbeat so that the heart is protected from damage while surgery is done to replace the valve with an artificial valve.

The artificial valve might be mechanical (made of man-made substances). Others are made out of animal tissue, often from a pig.

What to Expect After Surgery

You will recover in the hospital until you are healthy enough to go home. Depending on your overall health, you will likely go home a few days after surgery.

Surgery will likely involve a long recovery over several weeks. You will probably need to take 4 to 12 weeks off from work. It depends on the type of work you do and how you feel. In some cases, full recovery may take several months.

Types of valve replacement

- *Trans catheter aortic valve replacement*

  It does not require open-heart surgery. It is a minimally invasive procedure that uses catheters in blood vessels to replace the aortic valve with a specially designed artificial valve. The catheters are inserted through small cuts in the groin.

- *Aortic Valve Regurgitation*

Valve replacement surgery is the only cure for aortic valve regurgitation. It helps relieve symptoms and prevent heart failure. And it helps people live longer.

- *Aortic Valve Stenosis*

Valve replacement surgery is the only effective treatment for people who have severe aortic valve stenosis with symptoms. If you don't have surgery after you start having symptoms, you may die suddenly or develop heart failure. Surgery can help you have a more normal life span.

This procedure is available in a small number of hospitals. And it is not right for everyone. It might be done for a person who cannot have surgery or for a person who has a high risk of serious problems from surgery. For example, it might be an option if you are not healthy enough for an open-heart surgery.

Common, everyday tests given to determine heart disease

- Electrocardiogram (EKG) -- records the electrical activity of the heart and provides information about the rate and rhythm of the heart (painless and fast).
- The doctor may order a Holter monitor (Walkman-size device that you take home and record the activity of the heart over 24 hours-up to 1 week).
- Echocardiogram -- uses sound to provide a picture of the heart's structures. It can show enlarged heart, defects present at birth, or abnormal valves.

- X-Ray of the chest may show an enlarged heart or lung disease.
- If other conditions are suspected, blood and urine analysis may be needed.

LAUGHTER, THE BEST MEDICINE

From our wired fans & sisters on Facebook in answer to the question: *"Has anyone ever been told something funny or stupid relating to their devices?"*

Emma: I'm on my second battery, both of my scars have gone keloid, I've been told a few times I have lipstick on my chest! Why would I walk around with two lipstick kisses on my chest!!

Liz: A complete and total stranger once pointed at my pacer scar and asked me if I got stabbed. I looked at her with a straight face and said "Yes, in prison."

Rachel: My brother keeps saying he's going to get me a "Pacers" jersey...I'm his little Pacer.

Janie: I was misdiagnosed because my doc said I was way too young and fit to have anything that serious. I am 66! I guess I should feel flattered.

Dawn (me): I've been called "bionic" and the pacemaker is my "third boob." I've been told (not asked) "I'm sure your surgery will be no big deal, they just have to pop the battery out." (And you know....how???) "Can your pacemaker act as a garage door opener?" Or my biggest pet peeve: "So you can't use a microwave, right?"

Laurie: One person referred to my ICD as "your fake heart". LOL

Sherri: Why do they have to take the pacemaker out? They should just change the batteries. AND going for my yearly check, I always get asked if I'm going there to get my battery charged.

Tuffy: I always get "but you're so young!" Sometimes I feel like I disappointed them.

Mary: You're the energizer bunny now? I say no.....I am the Bionic Woman!!!! Gets them every time.

Arthur: I had someone tell me that I should wrap my chest in tin foil, because the NSA can track and record all of my conversations and movements using my pacemaker.

Helen: An elderly lady who had a friend with a pacemaker told me (before my first pm implant) that the procedure was 'just like having your ears pierced'. I wanted to grab her afterwards and ask who the heck pierced her ears.

Claudia: The "strangest" comment I have had was a person I knew suddenly went into a long story about a friend who died and the "pacemaker" kept trying to keep them alive.

Jennifer: I had just turned 25 when I got mine. My daughter was in kindergarten and told her teacher that her mom had gotten a pacemaker. So her teacher thought I was in my 60's. When she met me she said you're a lot younger than I thought.

Kerri: Always the same "at your age?" Like heart disease is only a senior special.

Mary E.: I went to the ER with kidney stones once. My pacemaker is located in my abdomen so it confuses a lot of people. A nurse came in after my imaging, pulled the curtain all secretly like, and whispered, "Do you have something implanted in you?" I was in too much pain to make a joke and just told her that it was my pm, but my dad said next time I need to say in shock, "That alien abduction was real?!!!" Hahaha!

Carla: I had a friend (new at the time) ask me in a disgusted voice why I'd want to show "that" off. (That being my scar.) Long story short, he thought it was a hickey at first glance and of course felt terrible when I explained what it was. Now its years later, hilarious to recall, and he's a brother to me.

Mark: "So, you can't use a microwave oven?"

MARIAN

Marian was so proud to say she was the very first member of WIRED4LIFE. On June 13, 2012 Marian passed away. It was a very sad day for our WIRED community. Marian was 89 years young, feisty and very independent. She was loving and so supportive of what I was trying to accomplish; way back in the beginning, when WIRED wasn't anything, just an idea on paper. Marian is the brightest star in the sky. xoxo

WIRED4LIFE

Facebook: http://www.facebook.com/wired4life

For kids: http://www.facebook.com/wired4lifekids

Website: http://www.wired4life.net

Our monthly newsletter is available for a yearly cost of $10.

For further information contact:

Dawn Huberty, WIRED4LIFE Founder
Email: dawnhuberty@wired4life.net

Thank you for taking the time to read my book, if you were inspired, please post a review on Amazon!

PS Please excuse grammatical mistakes.

WIRED4LIFE, My Journey to Becoming Wired by Dawn L. Huberty, revised September 2018

www.ingramcontent.com/pod-product-compliance
Lightning Source LLC
Chambersburg PA
CBHW051528170526
45165CB00002B/651